Complementary Therapies in Nursing and Midwifery

from vision to practice

Edited by
PAULINE McCABE

Foreword by
JUDY JACKA

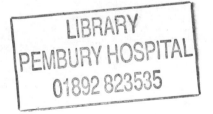

Ausmed Publications
Melbourne

Australasian Health Education Systems Pty Ltd
(ACN 005 611 626)
trading as
Ausmed Publications
277 Mount Alexander Road
ASCOT VALE, VICTORIA 3032, AUSTRALIA

First published March 2001

Further copies of this book and of all other Ausmed publications are available from the Distribution Manager, Ausmed Publications, PO Box 4086, Melbourne University, Victoria 3010, Australia.
Telephone +61 3 9375 7311.
Fax +61 3 9375 7299.
E-mail ausmed@ausmed.com.au
Home page www.ausmed.com.au

National Library of Australia Cataloguing-in-Publication data:

Complementary therapies in nursing and midwifery : from vision to practice.

Includes index
ISBN 0 9577988 1 4

1. Alternative medicine. 2. Nursing. 3. Midwifery. I. McCabe, Pauline. II.
Jacka, Judy, 1938-.
610.73

Edited by Trisha Dunning
Cover, design, typesetting and printing by Hyde Park Press, 5 Deacon Avenue, Richmond, South Australia 5033, telephone (08) 8234 2044, fax (08) 8234 1887, e-mail hpp@olis.net.au

Text set in 10/14 Garamond Book

Foreword

This is an exciting and timely book. It describes how nurses are pioneering complementary therapies within the medical system to give comfort and healing to their patients. It is 40 years since I graduated from general nursing training at Prince Henry's Hospital Melbourne with deep disappointment about the medical model of 1960. Perhaps my greatest concern was that nurses had insufficient opportunity and resources to give true caring to their patients. At that time there was little information about alternative medicine and healing in Australia, but my own quest gradually unfolded to include a world of healing that I experienced as truly remarkable. My goal became to create education that would combine natural therapies with a suitable standard of orthodox science and medicine. In 1997 the Victorian government accredited the Bachelor Degree in Health Science (Naturopathy) delivered by the Southern School of Natural Therapies, making it the first private college in Victoria to offer a government accredited complementary therapy course.

Therefore, during the last 30 years I have been intimately involved with practising natural therapies and the task of developing a degree standard course for training in the area. Throughout the 1980s many hundreds of nurses attended courses I conducted in natural therapies for the Council of Adult Education in Melbourne. Some of those nurses later enrolled to undertake training at our school. Indeed, since the birth of the school in 1961, nurses have featured strongly amongst our students and they have become excellent primary contact practitioners.

However, this book features nursing as a profession studying and developing research and guidelines about natural therapies that enhance nursing practice and improve patient care in a medical setting. It is now evident that nurses as a professional group want to know how to apply natural therapies to augment and improve the health of their patients within the current medical model. So, for me, this is an exciting book, because I now witness the educational and practice opportunities for complementary therapies that are taking place within the nursing profession. Perhaps this development will in time have powerful repercussions on the whole health care system. In a personal sense, my observations have come full circle, from those of a disillusioned graduate nurse, to observations of nurses creating opportunities to practise their own healing therapies.

While preparing to write this foreword it occurred to me that rarely have I heard much criticism directed towards nurses as a group, despite hearing harsh criticism of orthodox medicine from various directions. The nursing profession appears to have always created the perception of being a caring group that did the best for its patients despite all kinds of difficulties and challenges. It is, therefore, understandable that nurses are endeavouring to extend their practices to encompass therapies that they perceive as promoting a more human touch for their patients. In addition, research into the practices and therapies described in this book has demonstrated improved clinical outcomes in many of the patients concerned.

The book covers a wide range of areas that includes an historical perspective of natural therapies within the nursing profession; legal and ethical considerations; research possibilities and achievements; and educational considerations, as well as the pioneering experiences of nurses in areas such as nutrition, aromatherapy, massage, meditation, holistic coronary care, music therapy and the use of pet animals. The practice of complementary therapies within midwifery is an exciting development and what better way to give a child a peaceful start in life?

It is of interest that the term 'complementary therapies' rather than 'natural therapies' is used throughout the book. Educational and government committees dealing with such therapies have always been challenged to find the most appropriate label and definition of these healing arts and sciences. The therapies explored in this book are certainly those that can be seen to complement, rather than threaten orthodox medical practice. Hospital management could consider massage, aromatherapy, music and meditation as safe options compared, for instance, to the use of herbs and homeopathy.

I will be interested to observe how graduates from the double degree in nursing and naturopathy at Latrobe University and similar courses apply their training in herbal medicine and homeopathy in the workplace. Some authorities may view oral therapies as contradicting the use of pharmaceutical drugs. I look forward to a time when doctors will be versed sufficiently in herbal medicine and homeopathy to allow nurses trained in these specialities to augment or—dare I suggest it—replace the prescribed drug treatment in certain cases.

But these are thoughts for the future. This book is a brave and pioneering effort to show the current level of achievement by the nursing profession in using complementary therapies to date. Complementary therapies are obviously here to stay and patient demand is increasing as illustrated by the material in this book.

The appendices include current guidelines established by one state board and two federal nursing bodies with respect to complementary therapies and are therefore of particular interest. The impression gained from reading this section is that the nursing profession is taking a positive, creative and responsible position towards natural therapies. Indeed the whole book will be an inspiration to all nurses who wish to practise true healing arts within the medical workplace.

Judy Jacka ND, Grad Dip HRE
Retired Chairperson
Southern School of Natural Therapies
Melbourne, Australia

Contents

Figures

Tables

Dedication

Courage is not a word that is commonly applied to nurses in the context of professional development, however it needs to be acknowledged in those nurses who have begun to introduce complementary therapies into nursing practice. Nursing can be a conservative profession at times, and it takes a special kind of strength to introduce the new, particularly in an area that is still considered controversial by some of our colleagues in health care. The nurses who contributed to this book have all displayed the kind of professional courage needed at times to advance the profession, but in truth they represent only a tiny proportion of the many nurses who are working to integrate healing modalities into nursing practice. This book is dedicated to all nurses whose love of healing extends to the application of complementary therapies in conjunction with the therapeutic use of self. The development of complementary care in nursing not only supports the health and wellbeing of patients, it also has the potential to advance nursing practice, and to further define what nursing is.

Pauline McCabe

Acknowledgments

Ausmed Publications and the authors sincerely thank the following organisations and individuals for permission to reproduce the copyright material listed below:

- The Australian Nursing Federation policy statement: *Complementary and Alternative Therapies.* Appendix 1.
- The Royal College of Nursing, Australia position statement: *Complementary Therapies in Australian Nursing Practice.* Appendix 2.
- The Nurses Board of Victoria: *Guidelines for the Use of Complementary Therapies in Nursing Practice.* Appendix 3.
- The editors of *Diversity*, the magazine of The Australian Complementary Health Association. Sections of an article on therapeutic touch reproduced in Chapter 12.
- The Age newspaper, and the author, J Wright. Figure 14.1 in Chapter 14.
- Dr Wendy Moody, *Infection Control Guidelines for Animal-assisted Therapy in Hospitals,* which appears as an appendix to Chapter 14.
- The unknown author who wrote the Endnote to Chapter 14: *Things we can learn from a dog.*

Glossary of terms

DEFINITIONS

The definitions applied to natural therapies continue to be problematic and shifting, largely because they reflect how therapies are applied rather than specific types of therapies. A person may use any therapy in an alternative or complementary way, but generally speaking, developed systems of natural medicine such as naturopathy and traditional Chinese medicine tend to be more commonly used as alternatives because they can offer a developed theoretical perspective and a range of therapies. Nursing has the right, and indeed the obligation, to interpret natural therapies in the context of its own discipline, and is currently in the process of determining which natural therapies are complementary to its own role in health care. No doubt, as these therapies become integrated into practice and taught at undergraduate level, definitions will change again. For the moment, the definitions below reflect the contemporary situation.

Alternative medicine: Systems of health care such as naturopathy or traditional Chinese medicine which can be used either as an alternative or complementary to orthodox medicine.

Complementary care: Complementary care in nursing emphasises the centrality of caring and the healing role of the nurse, and recognises partnerships in health care that include the patient, the nurse, other health professionals, and the use of a wide range of interventions in the interests of health, healing, wellbeing and patient autonomy. Complementary care involves flexibility in the choice of therapy to provide the best outcome for the patient.

Complementary therapy: A range of natural therapies used to augment health, healing and wellbeing, complementing disease-focused medical treatment.

Holistic care: Recognises the whole person and their environment; understands that the nurse's action is never neutral, and that every action has an effect on the patient (Dossey et al., 1995). The holistic nurse therefore chooses to promote healing through therapeutic presence and appropriate interventions.

Healing: A process which moves towards reordering and reintegration of the bodymind. Healing can be either supported or suppressed, and incorporates the capacity to adapt where full healing is not possible, or to evolve to a higher level of wellness. Healing can potentially take place on some level of being until the moment of death (McCabe, 1995).

Natural therapy: Generic term for therapies which aim to promote health, healing and wellbeing by working to stimulate and support innate rebalancing and relaxation responses.

Nursing interventions: Nursing interventions are patient-centred interventions that are prescribed by nurses in response to nursing diagnoses and issues.

Preface

Complementary Therapies in Nursing and Midwifery—from vision to practice speaks to nurses and midwives about the integration of complementary therapies into practice. There are currently a number of books on complementary therapies in nursing and midwifery practice, but they generally place strong emphasis on describing specific therapies. The approach in this book is to bring to life for the reader the realities of attempting to integrate complementary therapies into practice. The book consists of three sections, which together cover issues of current interest, selected therapies, and examples of how complementary therapies were introduced into four different workplace settings. Consequently, there is a strong focus on areas that deal with professional, political and workplace concerns such as education, policy, research, and successful strategies for the introduction of complementary therapies. For the practitioner starting out, this book will provide the information needed to argue their case clearly and constructively; up-to-date references on research and significant articles; inspirational stories by nurses and midwives who have successfully pioneered the integration of complementary therapies; the strategies they used; ideas for beginners in research; useful tips for developing policy; clarification of legal concerns, and much more.

Complementary therapies in nursing and midwifery—from vision to practice will provide nurses and midwives interested in complementary care with essential background and current information concerning this exciting new area of interest. The book is divided into three sections. Section One covers the historical, political and professional issues relating to complementary therapies. Section Two discusses selected complementary therapies and Section Three gives examples of successful integration of complementary therapies in four practice settings.

Section One

Complementary therapies: historical, political and professional issues

The seven chapters in Section One cover a range of contemporary issues related to complementary therapies. The historical material in the first two chapters challenges notions of the relationship between complementary therapies, nursing and midwifery, and how the integration of complementary therapies into practice has the potential to significantly alter theory, practice, and the professional image of nursing and midwifery. Should complementary therapies be taught in undergraduate courses? These and other questions pertaining to education are covered, as well as concerns about legal and ethical issues. Research and evidence-based practice are assuming an increased role in practice. Issues around researching complex areas are discussed, and tips for getting started in clinical research are offered to beginning researchers. Finally, the potential career opportunities in complementary therapies and expanded practice in nursing and midwifery are discussed.

An overview of each chapter follows.

Chapter 1, **Nursing and complementary therapies: a natural partnership**, takes a chronological view of the relationship between nursing and natural therapies. Pauline McCabe, Senior Lecturer in Naturopathy at La Trobe University, begins with some historical insights into a relationship that can be traced back to Nightingale's era. The historical material is contrasted with the use of complementary therapies in contemporary, biomedically oriented health care. The integration of models grounded in the natural therapies paradigm will inevitably pose challenges in the future to our concepts of health, illness and healing, and some of these challenges are highlighted at the end of Chapter 1.

Chapter 2, **Complementary care: redefining nursing for the new millennium** by Jill Teschendorff, from the School of Nursing at Victoria University, discusses barriers to the implementation of complementary therapies into nursing practice. Internalised barriers derived from the power relationships within the health care system are the main focus of interest. These barriers are often overtly couched in a science versus non-science discourse that heavily influences nursing education, culture and practice. However, there are powerful covert barriers deeply embedded in the very construct of nursing's self-image, and these are revealed and challenged in this chapter. The integration of complementary therapies requires a cultural shift in the nursing and midwifery professions. Some suggestions on how integration can be achieved are provided.

Chapter 3, **Developing clinical practice guidelines,** deals with an issue of concern to many, the development of policies for the workplace. Trisha Dunning, a Clinical Nurse Consultant at St Vincent's Hospital in Melbourne and an aromatherapist, describes the process of developing complementary therapies guidelines for a large teaching hospital, commencing with a rationale for the use of guidelines. The development process and some of the difficulties encountered are described. The format and content areas of the policy are presented, along with a plan for evaluating its effectiveness.

Chapter 4, **Education and professional development**, is an expansive look at the history of healing and the way women's role and education have been defined through the centuries. Associate Professor Elaine Duffy of the Centre for Rural Health, Monash University, highlights a number of the issues and problems for nurses in the contemporary era regarding education in complementary therapies. New directions in CT education are demonstrated using various examples of innovative subjects and courses becoming available in undergraduate and postgraduate education.

Chapter 5, **Legal and ethical aspects of complementary therapies and complementary care,** was written by Judith Lancaster, a nurse and lawyer from the Faculty of Law at the University of Technology, Sydney. Judith provides comprehensive information about aspects of Australia's legal system that may influence the provision of complementary therapies by nurses, information that has been difficult for nurses to access in the past. The chapter covers how complementary therapies are regulated or self-regulated; liability; the nature of negligence; mechanisms for complaint by the public, and issues around consent.

Chapter 6, **Research issues in complementary therapies and holistic care**, provides a comprehensive discussion of the problems involved in researching complex areas of care. Professor Bev Taylor, Foundation Professor of Nursing at Southern Cross University, specialises in research of a holistic nature. Bev points out that complementary therapies and holistic nursing are not necessarily the same, and that different research approaches may be needed. The chapter provides a friendly introduction to research for those in the clinical area who may be interested in evaluating an aspect of nursing practice.

Chapter 7 is titled **Careers and opportunities: complementary therapies and future nursing.** As the title suggests, the chapter explores many interesting possibilities for nurses and midwives attracted to expanding their practice with complementary therapies. Sue Cechner combines her work as an aged care coordinator for the North Coast Region of New South Wales, with an independent practice as a nurse–natural therapist. The experience of synthesising these careers has given Sue considerable insight into career possibilities, that she shares with the reader.

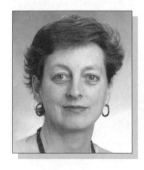

PAULINE McCABE
MHSc (PHC), RN, Midwife, ND, DipAc, MRCNA

Senior Lecturer in Naturopathy, School of Nursing, La Trobe University, Bundoora

Pauline McCabe has spent over thirty years in health care, and has qualifications in general nursing (Royal Melbourne Hospital 1969), acupuncture (Melbourne College of Acupuncture 1975), naturopathy (Southern School of Natural Therapies 1977), and midwifery (Queen Victoria Medical Centre 1979). Pauline's careers ran parallel for many years and then, much to her surprise, began to merge when she was asked to write a distance education unit on complementary therapies for nurses and midwives. A relationship with academia was established, leading to Master's and PhD projects, the latter still in progress. Pauline has made numerous contributions to the nursing literature on complementary therapies, including formulating national and state guidelines. She is currently Senior Lecturer in Naturopathy in the School of Nursing at La Trobe University, and is leading the design of a five year double degree in nursing and naturopathy that will be offered for the first time in 2001.

Nursing and complementary therapies: a natural partnership

Nurses and midwives need to be able to express their healing instincts. Too often the ideals of the beginning practitioner are put aside in the rush to comply with work practices. In spite of this the use of complementary therapies is increasing. Their use is not new in nursing or midwifery. This chapter will illustrate the natural partnership between nursing, midwifery and complementary therapies, drawing on historical and contemporary material. It asks the question: how might complementary therapies influence nursing theory and practice?, and looks at some of the challenges these therapies pose to nurses' understanding of illness and healing.

THE PAST

The history of nursing often focuses on Florence Nightingale and the professional, social and educational issues which so strongly influenced the evolution of early nursing. There is little interest in the interventions carried out by early nurses and midwives, activities now considered irrelevant. In the later part of the nineteenth century nursing was influenced by various natural therapies flourishing at the time. There was a strong popular backlash against orthodox medicine and its untrammelled use of toxic substances such as mercury, opium, and antimony. Medical theory held that disease had to be aggressively driven out by violent purging, sweating, salivation, bleeding and blistering (Griggs, 1982). There was little awareness of iatrogenic disease, so that when a patient died, as they often did, in grave distress, the death was attributed to the disease being too powerful for the treatment. Homoeopathy, osteopathy, nature cure, naturopathy, and North American herbal medicine all emerged to some extent in response to the injury and death perceived to be caused by orthodox treatments (Griggs, 1982).

A 'back to nature' movement emerged in Europe, and during the second half of the nineteenth century numerous sanatoria were established for treatment of the sick. A vegetarian diet, exercise, rest, hydrotherapy, fresh air, sunbathing, breathing exercises, positive thinking, prayer and fasting were among the therapies employed in the return to Hippocratic medicine which became known as nature cure. Germany and Austria were at the heart of this movement, and it was to Germany that Florence Nightingale travelled in 1851 to undertake nursing training. From her writings it appears that Nightingale's thinking was considerably influenced by nature cure philosophy, which espoused a vitalistic approach to healing and health promotion, and the need to work with nature to achieve a cure (McCabe, 2000a).

Around the turn of the century, natural therapists of various disciplines rivalled orthodox practitioners in popularity, particularly in the United States (Griggs, 1982). Homoeopathic hospitals were established in many cities (Melbourne and Sydney each had one), and there was increasing popular interest in the treatment of disease by natural methods. One of the best known nature cure hospitals in the United States was the Battle Creek Sanatorium, which provided rest cures, rehabilitation after acute infectious disease, and emergency surgery. In this environment, nursing theory and practice were largely related to the use of nature cure therapies.

In 1893 Mrs SM Baker, matron of the Battle Creek Sanatorium, spoke at the world's first international nursing conference in Chicago. Baker's paper gives a fascinating insight into the work of nurses in a hospital with a nature cure philosophy (most hospitals at the time followed orthodox medical principles). She comments that 'the rational medicine of the present day is requiring less of drugs and more of natural remedies' (Baker, in Hampton 1949:194).

One of the principal therapies was nutrition. Diets were individually prescribed and patients were taught the principles of a healthy, whole food diet. Massage, active and passive exercises, fresh air, sunbathing and breathing exercises were all used. Electrotherapy, the use of mild electrical currents, was popular for its apparent relaxing and vitalising effects (a modern version is used by physiotherapists today). Baker considered hydrotherapy, the therapeutic use of hot and cold water, the most advantageous nursing intervention. Enemas, compresses, baths, mineral waters and fomentations are all types of hydrotherapy. The application of moist heat and cold to different parts of the body was used to achieve many things, including reducing fever and inflammation, pain relief and relaxation.

Speaking at the Chicago Congress Baker said:

> *How few, outside of the trained profession, understand that of the different forms of hydropathic treatment, one will produce a tonic effect, another a sedative, another a moderate eliminative, another a full eliminative effect; that one will diminish pelvic congestion, another will reduce cerebral congestion, and so on through the list of ailments and remedial measures. The relief from pain which a hot sitz-bath and foot-bath will give, the invigorating effect of a cool shallow bath, the soothing influence of the hot spray, or alternate hot and cold sponging of the spine, the comfort of a blanket-pack or home-arranged Turkish bath in conditions requiring their use, or of the cool wet-sheet pack in fevers, the indescribable exhilaration of a salt glow are something known only to those who have witnessed their magic working.*

(Baker, 1893)

The health and happiness of nurses was also a consideration, and they were given advice to exercise and have regular massage to build strength and a calm disposition. Happiness came from working in Battle Creek's healing environment where, unlike the public hospital system with its limited funds and time constraints, a wider range of interventions was available and nurses had a more personalised relationship with their patients. Access to training and experience in natural therapies, and active contribution to the healing process, were found to increase personal and professional satisfaction.

Florence Nightingale, speaking at the same Congress as Baker, discussed the nature of health and sickness, in the context of classic nature cure theory:

> *Sickness or disease is nature's way of getting rid of the effects of conditions which have interfered with health. It is nature's attempt to cure. (The aim of nursing is to put the person) in the best possible conditions for nature to restore or to preserve health ....*

(Nightingale, in Hampton 1949:26).

Her words echo the need to work with nature, rather than against it, if we wish to assist the healing process—a philosophy instinctively followed by Australia's most famous nurse–natural therapist, Sister Elizabeth Kenny. Many readers will be familiar with Kenny's treatment of polio or infantile paralysis in the Queensland epidemic of 1911. As a young, untrained, practical nurse working alone in an isolated rural area, Kenny was called to visit a child in agony with severe cramps. Kenny telegraphed a description to a local doctor. The return message said 'Infantile paralysis. No known treatment. Do the best you can with the symptoms presenting themselves' (in Cohn,

1975:41). Polio was relatively unknown in Australia in 1911. Kenny had some experience with muscle spasm and the use of exercise in strengthening frail muscles, and was unaware of the medical treatment of infantile paralysis—forcibly straightening and splinting the legs.

Kenny applied her knowledge to the child acutely ill with polio. The obvious treatment was heat. Hot salt packs were ineffective so Kenny turned to hydrotherapy, using strips of woollen blanket wrung out in hot water and wrapped around the twisted limbs. The relief was immediate, encouraging nurse and parents to keep up the treatment for several days until the acute phase was over. The little patient walked again, as did many others Kenny later treated for polio, including the former Queensland Premier Sir Joh Bjelke-Petersen. However, Kenny's treatment was rejected by the medical profession, and the struggle to win recognition of her management of polio lasted several decades.

THE PRESENT

For most of this century the quiet benefits of natural therapies have been eclipsed by the enthralling drama of medical progress. The virtues of modern medicine have shone, while its failures are all too often obscured from public view. Nurses, perhaps more than most people, are aware of both the benefits and the shortcomings of a technological, disease-oriented system of health care. Some achievements of modern medicine, such as treatment of severe trauma or birth defects, border on the miraculous. Nevertheless, the great bulk of the patient population suffers from so-called lifestyle diseases such as respiratory, musculoskeletal and cardiovascular problems, and the complications of ongoing pharmaceutical management.

Consequently, there has been a tremendous increase in the use and availability of complementary therapies in Western countries in recent decades. The increased utilisation of complementary therapies has coincided with the rapid medicalisation of health, and an unprecedented rise in technological approaches to disease. Concerns about the effects of medical care on consumers, the health care system, and the economies of both wealthy and poor nations are well documented. In Australia, the response to escalating health care costs has been a 'slash and burn' economic rationalism which has affected all sectors of health care, and nursing in particular. Yet in spite of punishing workloads, decreased funding, and scepticism from colleagues, more and more nurses are finding ways of incorporating complementary therapies into patient care.

Nurses are consumers as well as being the largest group of health care providers, and they participate with the general population in using and learning about complementary therapies. Patients are increasingly consulting natural therapists for a wide range of problems (Lloyd et al., 1993), and generally consider them to be effective practitioners (Kermode et al., 1999). About 50% of the Australian population uses some form of natural therapy, spending, in 1993, approximately $621 million on remedies and $309 million on consultations, compared to the $360 million contributed by patients to the pharmaceutical benefits scheme (MacLennan et al., 1996).

Oral vitamins, herbs or minerals are purchased over the counter by around 60% of Australians, with herbal products showing the fastest growth in sales (Scherer, Australia, 1998). Significantly, many people create their own form of complementary care by attending both medical practitioners and natural therapists at the same time (Lloyd et al., 1993). People choose complementary therapies for various reasons. Apart from concern about the side effects of drugs, short consultations, and the limited range of treatment options available from medical practitioners, clients are looking for better patient–practitioner interaction and a more holistic approach to the causes and treatment of ill health (Hunter, 1997).

Aggressive and harmful medical treatments, and the lack of a proactive approach to healing and wellbeing, support a system where outcomes are often measured in terms of morbidity and mortality. An Australian study by the National Health Strategy (1992) found that drug related problems and adverse reactions due to misuse, inappropriate prescribing, and unavoidable reactions contributed to 30 000–40 000 hospital admissions and 700–900 deaths. The estimated cost of adverse drug reactions in 1992 was $68–87 million. The elderly are particularly at risk. Of those older people living in the community, 17.9% used more than 26 prescriptions in a six-month period. In contrast, 34% of those in residential care facilities used more than 26 prescriptions in six months. Fifty-four percent of residents in aged care facilities were prescribed drugs inappropriately at least once in a six-month period (National Health Strategy, 1992).

Nursing is closely allied to medicine, and the increasingly expensive and mechanistic approach of the biomedical model may have precipitated a move towards nursing's espoused holistic approach (Trevelyan and Booth,1994; and Dossey et al.,1995). An increasing number of nurses in Australia and other developed countries are adopting complementary therapies in their practice, either as an adjunct to traditional care or as the predominant therapy (McCabe et al., 1995; Rankin-Box, 1995a; Dossey et al., 1995; Cole and Shanley, 1998; and James, 1999). Nursing theory also supports the use of complementary therapies. Martha Rogers' work, grounded in new physics, supports the existence of a human energy field and the irreducible nature of human beings (Rogers, 1990).

A wider interpretation of health, which incorporates the lifestyle patterns that contribute to illness, broadens both nursing diagnosis and interventions (Newman, 1987). Knowledge of human behaviour and needs assists nurses to promote health and healing and advance nursing care and interventions that complement medical care (Watson, 1985). Transcultural nursing (Leininger, 1991) highlights the need to respect cultural beliefs and practices surrounding health, an approach which can be extended to those who value natural therapies. In Australia, various state registration boards and professional associations have developed guidelines for use of complementary therapies in nursing, for example the Royal College of Nursing, Australia (1997) and the Nurses Board of Victoria (1999).

There is no published data available in Australia about the extent of the use of complementary therapies by nurses, their level of competence or the types of therapies they employ. However, anecdotal evidence points to considerable interest in, and increasing use of, complementary therapies by nurses, particularly in aged care, palliative care, critical care and midwifery (McCabe, 1996). Some private complementary therapy colleges report informally that up to 25% of their students are nurses (Borland, 1999).

THE FUTURE

The use of complementary therapies has the potential to revolutionise nursing theory and practice and, in consequence, the Australian health care system. This may seem a rather grand speculation, yet complementary therapies have already markedly changed the profile of health care in the broad private sector. The question is: what kind of changes might complementary therapies make to the discipline of nursing in the coming years? The therapies themselves are an entry point for what may become deeper conceptual changes to the understanding of health and healing.

The principles of complementary therapies

Most of the theoretical frameworks for complementary therapies have been developed as models that represent a holistic understanding and experience of bodymind, health and healing, which is somewhat different from the contemporary interpretation as body-mind-spirit-environment. Nurses who have qualified in a complementary therapy and are applying it in a nursing context are likely to be conceptualising use according to some, or all of the following broadly stated principles:

- The human bodymind has an innate drive towards healing and adaptation. Treatment and care should support this process as far as is possible.
- Energy is vital to the system's capacity to reorder itself. Treatment and care should increase vitality, not deplete it.
- Treat the whole person. Health and disorder are the outcomes of complex and interacting physical, personal, social and environmental factors.
- Disease is an entirety that affects the whole person and presents as a pattern or patterns. All signs, symptoms and sensations are relevant.
- Find the cause. Treatment cannot be effective unless the underlying cause and predisposing factors are addressed.
- Do no harm. Wherever possible use therapies which support the individual's healing capacity.
- Educate the patient. The practitioner has a responsibility to educate the patient regarding lifestyle factors which may contribute to ill health.
- Support dignity and quality of life for patients in the terminal phase of life.

(Adapted from Pizzorno, 1996).

Many of these principles have strong parallels in nursing theory and practice, which partly explains why complementary therapies fit so well into nursing and midwifery. Complementary therapies have not commanded the attention of many nurse academics to date. As the use of complementary therapies increases and new models of care emerge complementary therapies will command the attention of theorists interested in researching concepts as well as therapy outcomes. The stories at the beginning of the chapter raise a number of conceptual issues which mark part of the boundary between traditional natural therapy thinking and contemporary understandings of the body, health and illness. Some of these issues are raised below.

THE PURPOSEFUL ASPECT OF ILLNESS

In natural therapies the signs and symptoms of illness are understood to result from a combination of the effects of pathological factors and the innate responses to those factors. Innate responses include white cell activity, fever, and elimination of toxins (sweat, diarrhoea, pus, etc.), activities that are aided by vitality, the adequacy of available nutrients, and mental-emotional support for the body's healing work (McCabe, 2000b). The purpose of these responses is to restore balance (Pizzorno, 1996; and Jacka, 1998). Their very nature indicates the type of imbalance present and suggests ways to assist the bodymind's re-balancing efforts. Where a full return to prior normality is not possible the system will adapt and survive the best way it can, often with annoying ongoing symptoms.

CHOOSING SUPPORTIVE THERAPIES

Complementary therapies work from the perspective of assisting healing and wellbeing. They require an approach to disorder that comprehends the purposive nature of many symptoms, and allows the practitioner to work with the bodymind, listening and responding to its messages. Accurate differentiation between disease process and adaptive or re-balancing responses is essential. Treatment should both manage the disease process and strengthen and support the bodymind in its efforts to regain balance, and should do no harm.

EDUCATE OR BLAME?

Disease is often described as accidental, unfair and meaningless. Such an interpretation allows suppression of symptoms and 'protects' the patient from the knowledge that prior lifestyle may have contributed to the evolution of the disease. This approach avoids the accusation that one is 'blaming the victim'. However, education can be undertaken in a way that supports the person, interprets the disease as expressing meaningful indicators to improved health and wellbeing, and acknowledges the difficulties of remaining healthy in a society that condones many disease-inducing practices.

RE-BALANCING RATHER THAN SUPPRESSION

When certain signs and symptoms are understood as purposeful efforts to restore balance or to adapt, it is not logical to suppress them unless they are out of control or life threatening. For example, diarrhoea due to food poisoning is largely an attempt to eliminate poisons and the body needs to do that. However if dehydration is a threat, gentle re-balancing rather than suppression would be the preferred response. Treatment might include, for example, fluid replacement, slippery elm powder to protect the gut wall from irritation, rest, temporary fasting, and later yoghurt to help replace lost normal gut flora. Elimination of toxins and re-balancing of normal function is the aim, rather than suppressing the diarrhoea and retaining toxins in the gut. In a different scenario, treatment aims for the dying person might include palliation, re-balancing or suppression. Complementary care always demands the ability to move flexibly, and appropriately, from one paradigm to another.

RE-BALANCE AND REHABILITATION

The concept of re-balancing is very different from cure (Watson, 1985). The latter commonly involves removal of a problem via surgery or ongoing management with drugs, where attention to contributing lifestyle factors may be overlooked. Re-balancing considers ways to support a return to healthy, balanced function, an approach advocated by nursing theory. Natural therapies, theory and practice, offer a range of models that can challenge nursing to reinterpret mindbody function, and foster a proactive role in healing and the restoration of balance. Once the need for any medical stabilisation is past, aged care and recovering clients are particularly suited to re-balancing interventions from nursing.

THE IMPORTANCE OF NUTRITION AND ELIMINATION

Many common illnesses are understood in natural therapies to originate from an unsuitable diet that results in dysfunction of the stomach, intestines, liver, gall bladder, and pancreas. Nutritional research increasingly validates this stance. The concept of elimination in complementary therapies is also broader than the contemporary orthodox understanding. The function of bowels, bladder, skin and lungs is evident externally, but the daily drainage of the waste products of metabolism, drugs, pathogens and pollutants from the cells is internal and adds to the burden carried by the liver, blood, lymphatic drainage and the immune system. Elimination can be encouraged by the consumption of fluids and fibre, but also by exercise, massage, deep breathing, and a plentiful supply of the nutrients, herbs and foods employed in detoxification and elimination (Carper, 1988; and Jacka,1998). Many chronic diseases and recurring disorders can be assisted by attention to nutrition and elimination. Nurses are in an excellent position to advise clients about dietary modification (see Chapter 8). Dietary education is one of the strongest means of empowering people with regard to ongoing healing and health management.

ASSESSMENT AND DIAGNOSIS

There is clearly an integral relationship between nursing assessment, diagnosis, and prescription of nursing interventions (Snyder, 1992). Whatever system of nursing diagnosis is used, it must link to the prescribed interventions to enable a systematic and rational approach to care. Complementary therapy interventions must relate to nursing assessment, have a demonstrated rationale for use and be documented in the care plan. These actions will also facilitate evaluation of the outcomes.

THE FUNCTIONAL PERSPECTIVE

Complementary therapies have the potential to integrate with holistic nursing assessment because traditionally complementary therapies, like nursing diagnosis, take a functional and pattern-oriented perspective. In nursing this is defined as assessment of the normal or characteristic performance of an individual, and incorporates physical, mental, emotional and social functions (Barkauskas et al., 1998). However, in the natural therapies, functional diagnosis closely follows the manifestations of disorder. Patterns of dysfunction familiar to the natural therapies are identified, then matched to an appropriate remedy such as a herb or essential oil. The properties and actions of plants have been recognised for centuries, and research frequently supports traditional usage based on centuries of clinical experience (Claus and Tyler, 1965). Chamomile, for example, has relaxant and anti-inflammatory properties, fennel is an expectorant, and ginger and peppermint are carminatives. Aromatherapy has incorporated many of the traditional uses of plants into its repertory.

It is important to realise that describing dysfunction is different from naming a disorder, for example a functional assessment of headache would describe the type of pain and any factors associated with it. A spasmodic headache emanating from the shoulder and neck muscles may respond to relaxing massage. A full throbbing headache associated with fever will usually ease with cooling of the body and feet. A dull congestive headache associated with a cold may need warming stimulants such as ginger and garlic to loosen mucus. Specific measures to apply depend on the therapy to be used and the practitioner's level of skill in assessment and use of particular treatments. A full description of signs, symptoms and associated factors clearly reveals the dysfunction, facilitates the choice of therapeutic intervention and the rationale for that choice, and enables documentation and evaluation.

POTENTIAL FOR DISUSE SYNDROME: A CASE STUDY

A person presenting with partial paralysis of the right arm and leg following recent stroke, and early signs of foot drop and closure of the hand, is having physiotherapy but requires additional support. Nursing assessment reveals muscle weakness, cold limbs, poor reflexes, discomfort, anxiety and limited movement, all indications for massage. The aims of complementary therapy treatment therefore, are to improve muscle strength and responsiveness, increase circulation, promote movement, reduce discomfort, and provide caring touch. Nursing interventions could include a ten-minute massage of the right limbs every four hours, gentle rotation of the joints, passive movements and daily back massage. Some of these parameters are measurable.

EXTENDING THE ROLE OF NURSING CARE

The role of primary care is increasingly becoming the domain of nurses and midwives, for example in aged care or remote area nursing. In recent years complementary therapy nursing interventions have mainly been used for relaxation and to enhance wellbeing but increasingly, the value of complementary therapies for treating minor functional problems is being acknowledged (Trevelyan and Booth, 1994; and Cole and Shanley, 1998). A person may experience many uncomfortable symptoms apart from the signs and symptoms that are attributable to a disease. Problems such as diarrhoea, constipation, insomnia, itching, nausea, cramps, aching muscles, fatigue, headache, anxiety, misery, flushing, dry skin, indigestion, sadness, cough, or menstrual pain, often 'fall through the cracks' of medical care, being regarded as too insignificant to treat. These problems frequently become nursing problems, for which complementary therapies offers a range of non-pharmaceutical options. The potential for reducing drug intake, especially in elderly people and pregnant women, needs to be explored (see Section Three).

The extended role of the nurse or midwife may take two forms: first, increasing uptake of medical tasks with attendant mechanisation of nursing care; and second, a return to core values with client-centred care, professionalism, and attention to the therapeutic power of nursing (Cole and Shanley, 1998). Complementary care is more aligned with the latter, embracing an extended role centred in holistic nursing, an active nurse–client partnership, and integration of complementary therapies into standard care, health promotion and healing.

STRATEGIES FOR INTRODUCING COMPLEMENTARY THERAPIES

Judging from my own conversations with nurses interested in complementary therapies, and from the anecdotal evidence suggesting there are large numbers of nurses with qualifications in complementary therapies who are not utilising them in nursing practice, barriers to their implementation and utilisation remain significant (O'Connor, 1997). These barriers largely centre around adherence to the medical model, resistance to taking up a full professional role, and concerns regarding evidence. All of these issues will be covered in later chapters of this book.

Many nurses feel too isolated and disempowered to implement complementary therapies, but there are a number of strategies that will foster success. Initially, it may be helpful to read the literature about change and resistance thereto (Rankin-Box, 1995b).

The strategies used by the authors in Section Three of this book provide practical examples of how some nurses have negotiated change. Finally, the following list of strategies may provide ideas for a starting point.

- Seek like-minded colleagues and form an interest group. Contact nurses and midwives who have successfully introduced complementary therapies to other workplaces.
- Gather information, articles, guidelines, policies, and research.
- Gain qualifications in a therapy of interest or enlist the services of an independent practitioner.
- Create clear and achievable objectives.
- Hold information/poster sessions to explain the complementary therapy and its relationship to nursing and medical practice.
- Involve relevant stakeholders, particularly supporters in management and consumer representatives. Collect patient feedback/surveys.
- Consider relevant professional issues such as quality control, ethical and legal issues, public demand, policy development, insurance, education and evaluation.
- Debate the relationship between nursing or midwifery, complementary therapies and medical practice. Learn to argue your case using established research and theory, for example, holistic nursing, effects of complementary therapies on reducing stress and pain, and role of nurses and midwives in promoting healing, health and wellbeing.
- Seek out colleagues who are resistant and get their help to identify areas of concern, and how they may be overcome.
- Start simply by creating a healing environment wherever possible. Introduce colour, quiet time, relaxation sessions, healing music, exercise, aromatherapy, humorous and educational videos (McCabe, 1998; and James, 1999).

CONCLUSION

The potential for healing is built into the very fabric of our being. The work required to achieve it is often slow, practical, and thorough, requiring time and patience. It is not the stuff of television drama, but a gift of nature innate within each person. Natural therapies look at the same suffering but through a different lens, and their traditions, often based on centuries of experience, reflection and experiment, offer models of theory and assessment from which nursing can potentially learn much. Like nursing, their skills are functional and clinical but they teach the practitioner to examine closely the behaviour of the bodymind, relating part to whole, and using information from all the senses to describe its patterns and processes fully and accurately. The problem of evaluation in complementary therapies is real, but not insurmountable. It applies not only to the effects of therapies, but to the assessment upon which those interventions are based. Critical thinking and reflection, long the tools of genuine healers, will remain vital to any care that embraces the complexity of being.

REFERENCES

Baker SM (1893-1949): Nursing in Homes, Private Hospitals and Sanitariums. In: Hampton IA (ed.) (1949): *Nursing of the Sick 1893.* New York: McGraw-Hill: 191–201.

Barkauskas V, Stoltenberg-Allen K, Baumann L, Darling-Fisher C (1998): *Health and Physical Assessment.* St Louis: Mosby.

Borland M (1999): Increased recognition of natural medicine. *Nursing Review.* July, p.12.

Carper J (1988): *The Food Pharmacy.* London: Simon and Schuster.

Claus EP, Tyler VE (1965): *Pharmacognosy* (5th ed). Philadelphia: Lea and Febiger.

Cohn V (1975): *Sister Kenny: the Woman who Challenged the Doctors.* Minneapolis; University of Minnesota Press.

Cole A, Shanley E (1998): Complementary therapies as a means of developing the scope of professional nursing practice. *Journal of Advanced Nursing.* 27:1171–1174.

Dossey B, Keegan L, Guzzetta K, Kolkmeier L (1995): *Holistic Nursing: a Handbook for Practice* (2nd ed). Gaithersburg, MD: Aspen Publishers.

Griggs B (1982): *Green Pharmacy: a History of Herbal Medicine.* London: Norman and Hobhouse.

Hunter A (1997): Why do people see natural therapists? A review of the surveys. *Diversity.* 10:15–19.

Jacka J (1998): *A-Z of Natural Therapies* (revised edition). Melbourne: Lothian.

James K (1999): The joys and pitfalls of complementary therapies. *Australian Nursing Journal.* 6 (8):34.

Kermode S, Myers S, Ramsay L (1999): Using natural and complementary therapies on NSW's North Coast: results from a new survey. *Diversity.* 16:13–17.

Leininger M (ed.) (1991): *Culture, Care, Diversity and Universality: a Theory of Nursing.* New York: National League for Nursing.

Lloyd P, Lupton D, Wiesner D, Hasleton S (1993): Choosing alternative therapy: an exploratory study of sociodemographic characteristics and motives of patients resident in Sydney. *Australian Journal of Public Health.* 17 (2):135–144.

MacLennan AH, Wilson DH, Taylor AW (1996): Prevalence and cost of alternative medicine in Australia. *The Lancet.* March 2, 347:569–573

McCabe P (1996): *Nursing and Complementary Therapies: the Promotion of Healing, Health and Wellbeing.* In: Taylor B (ed.): *Complementary Therapies in Australian Nursing Practice.* Deakin, ACT: Royal College of Nursing, Australia.

McCabe P (1998): Complementary therapies as nursing interventions: rationale for use and strategies for integration. Paper presented at Complementary Therapies and Pain, Ausmed Publications Seminar, 17 March, Melbourne.

McCabe P (2000a): Naturopathy, Nightingale, and nature cure: a convergence of interests. *Complementary Therapies in Nursing and Midwifery.* 6 1:4–8.

McCabe P (2000b): Unpublished Doctoral thesis.

McCabe P, Ramsay L, Taylor B 1995: Complementary therapies in relation to nursing practice in Australia: Discussion paper No. 2. Deakin ACT: Royal College of Nursing, Australia.

National Health Strategy 1992: Issues in pharmaceutical drug use in Australia. Melbourne: Issues Paper No 4.

Newman M (1987): *Nursing's Emerging Paradigm: the Diagnosis of Pattern.* In: McLane AM (ed.) *Classification of Nursing Diagnosis.* Proceedings of the seventh conference, North American Nursing Diagnosis Association, St Louis: CV Mosby.

Nightingale F (1893–1949): *Sick Nursing and Health Nursing.* In: Hampton IA (ed.) (1949): *Nursing of the Sick* 1893. New York: McGraw-Hill, pp. 24–43.

Nurses Board of Victoria (1999): *Guidelines for Use of Complementary Therapies in Nursing Practice* (2nd ed). Melbourne: Nurses Board of Victoria.

O'Connor J (1997): Nursing and natural therapies: barriers to implementation. *Australian Journal of Holistic Nursing.* 4 (1):24–31.

Pizzorno J (1996): Chapter 12, Naturopathic Medicine. In: Micozzi MS (ed) *Fundamentals of Complementary and Alternative Medicine.* New York: Churchill Livingstone.

Rankin-Box D (ed) (1995a): *The Nurses' Handbook of Complementary Therapies.* New York: Churchill Livingstone.

Rankin-Box D (1995b): Managing Change in the Workplace. In: Rankin-Box D (ed.) *The Nurses' Handbook of Complementary Therapies.* New York: Churchill Livingstone.

Rogers M (1990): Nursing: Science of Unitary, Irreducible, Human Beings: Update 1990. In: Barrett EAM, *Visions of Rogers' Science-Based Nursing.* New York: National League for Nursing.

Royal College of Nursing, Australia (1997): Position Statement: *Complementary Therapies in Australian Nursing Practice.* Deakin, ACT: Royal College of Nursing, Australia.

Scherer Australia (1998): Vitamins, minerals, herbals and health supplements: usage data. Melbourne: RP Scherer Australia.

Snyder M (1992): *Independent Nursing Interventions* (2nd ed). Albany, NY: Delmar.

Trevelyan J, Booth B (1994): *Complementary Medicine for Nurses, Midwives and Health Visitors.* London: Macmillan Press.

Watson J (1985) *Nursing: Human Science and Human Care.* Connecticut: Appleton-Century-Crofts.

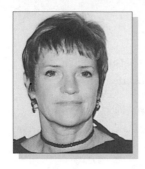

JILL TESCHENDORFF
RN, Midwife, MCHN, B App Science, MHsc, Cert Massage

School of Nursing, Victoria University of Technology

With extensive nursing experience in paediatrics, midwifery, maternal and child health and general nursing, Jill has a strong interest in facilitating change through research and teaching. A qualified massage therapist, Professor Teschendorff believes that complementary health care offers nurses the opportunity to implement effective, practical care that is holistic and under the control of nurses. Her research interests are broad and they include overseas skills recognition in Australia, intercultural communication, cultural adjustments of migrant nurses and the effects of massage on post-operative pain. She is currently investigating the health beliefs that impact on the practice of massage. Professor Teschendorff has extensive experience in the accreditation of courses in complementary health care and was a member of the advisory committee for the Review of *Guidelines for Use of Complementary Therapies in Nursing Practice* for the Nurses Board of Victoria.

Complementary care: redefining nursing for the new millennium

INTRODUCTION

The growth in the complementary health care industry has been enormous in the last few years. With an increasing demand for well qualified practitioners, education and training (traditionally the domain of private providers) is now offered within the TAFE and higher education sector. Anecdotal evidence suggests that a sizeable percentage of students undertaking study in this field are nurses (McCabe, 1994; and McCabe et al., 1995). However, despite the number of nurses with qualifications in complementary therapies, there is little evidence to suggest that complementary health care is an integral part of nursing education, or that complementary therapies are commonly used by nurses within mainstream health care[1]. The reasons for this are not clear, but it is postulated that barriers such as the medically dominated health care hierarchy and the socialisation of the nursing workforce are critical factors.

The number of nurses who practise complementary therapies in Australia is unknown. In Victoria, Bonawitt and Evans (1994) conducted a study of 130 nurses in independent, private and fee-for-service practice, and over half of the participants were complementary nurse therapists. The study found that only 19% of independent/private nurses practice in institutional settings. Anecdotal evidence indicates that nurses who have trained in complementary therapies practice professionally outside the institutional setting, or utilise their skills with family and friends. This suggests that nurses recognise the need for a new approach to health care delivery. Nevertheless, for a number of reasons they[2] may be reluctant to incorporate complementary health care into their practice.

THE NEED FOR A NEW MODEL OF CARE

There is growing concern in nursing circles about the increasing focus on technological and pharmacological approaches to health care. As medical interventions become increasingly sophisticated many of the traditional carative practices take second place to the imperatives imposed by the mechanised implementation of care (George and Davis, 1998). Application of the biomedical model has resulted in nursing being 'captive to . . . a medical system whose goal is to cure acute diseases rather than to improve quality of life' (Allan and Hall, 1988: 33). A further concern for nurses is the high rate of iatrogenesis. The biomedical model is a highly interventionist approach to health care which may result in short or long-term damage to the patient[3].

The situation has frustrated many nurses who find they spend a great deal of their time 'nursing the equipment' and have little time to focus on the patient. Allan and Hall (1988:33) point out that 'The time is overdue to move away from the technological imperative and toward holistic models that have as their major focus a concern with people's lives'. Complementary health care offers this opportunity, but there are social and structural barriers to its implementation that must first be recognised and overcome. One significant factor is the socialisation of nurses.

THE SOCIALISATION OF NURSES

The spiralling cost of health care together with recent savage budget cuts and subsequent 'downsizing' of the work force have impacted heavily on nurses, the largest professional group in the health industry. The beleaguered nurses who remain in the workforce must cope with a greatly increased workload, complicated by the demands of a highly mechanised work place. This burden is exacerbated by the constant stress that nurses experience when caring for people who are in physical or psychological crisis.

Faced with the threat of the unknown people often cling to familiar rituals and routines for comfort and reassurance. The seminal work of Isobel Menzies in 1970 studied the responses of nurses to their extremely stressful occupation. Although Menzies' study was conducted nearly 30 years ago, the results are still relevant and throw some light on nurses' socialised resistance to change.

Working with people who are ill or facing major life changes, nurses must cope with the psychological stress of patients and family, and more significantly, their own fears about suffering and death. Menzies (1970) found nurses developed a range of distancing behaviours and practices, which will be all too familiar to the reader, in order to cope with the stress that other people's suffering provokes. Adhering to tasks which reduce or restrict contact with patients, nurses standardise care so that all patients are treated as if they are the same. The result is a strict adherence to routines and rituals.

Nurses also distance themselves from patients by their detached behaviour and avoiding expressions of emotion. The perpetuation of conformity through standardising the ward environment and wearing uniforms is another convention that reinforces distance. In addition, decision making is avoided by 'routinising' care, thus avoiding the possibility of making the 'wrong' decision. When a final judgement is made, checking and counter checking is carried out to dissipate the anxiety that may result. Finally, the maintenance of a rigid hierarchy ensures the delegation of ultimate responsibility to superiors.

These behaviours may throw some light on the guarded interest in complementary therapies and their implementation into nursing care. The standardisation of nursing care, adherence to routines and rituals and avoidance of decision making, may result in nurses being reluctant to initiate new therapeutic approaches to care, irrespective of their efficacy and the nurse's competence. Newness is generally greeted with suspicion within the realms of nursing practice. Distancing and de-personalising behaviours are in direct contradiction to the person-centred approach of many complementary therapies, where the nurse-therapist facilitates the innate healing powers of the client through the 'therapeutic use of self'. This approach requires close personal interaction between the giver and receiver of care and acceptance of responsibility. These concepts are discussed elsewhere in the book.

This conservative nursing social system mitigates anxiety but it also stands in the way of change. In particular, it obstructs nurse-initiated, nurse-directed care. However, an equally potent barrier to change is the power relationships within the health care system that affect the degree to which nurses maintain control over their practice.

THE POWER RELATIONSHIPS WITHIN THE HEALTH CARE SYSTEM

Organisations in health care are bounded by history, culture, politics and the socio-economic climate (Taylor, 1997). The power relationships within the health care system severely limit the autonomy of nurses, and the implementation of change by nurses (even in the area of nursing care) is extremely difficult. Duckett (1984:959–966) identifies three principle structural interests in the struggle for power within the health care system; the professional monopolists (medicine), the corporate rationalists (the health bureaucracy), and the equal health advocates. Nurses, despite their numbers, do not exercise significant power, and although nursing is central to health care, to a large degree the control of patient care is in the hands of medicine and management. Added to this is the current economic imperative to contain costs and increase productivity. As Grace (1990) points out, nurses must find ways to promote and maintain humanistic nursing care and at the same time employ the parsimonious principles applied to running an efficient business.

In a treatment system primarily concerned with curing illness through the use of pharmacology and advanced technology, the nursing qualities of caring and supporting are not seen as critical to the scientific curative process. Nursing knowledge and nursing care are seen as inferior to medical management, scientific knowledge and cure, and yet nursing is central to medical practice (Jolley and Brykczynska, 1993:45). The dominance of the biomedical model has reduced or impeded the power and legitimacy of other less disease oriented professions, including nursing and complementary health care. Attempts by nurses to break into the economic and political monopoly have generally been unsuccessful; the two clear examples being independent nurse practitioners and midwives. However, the medical monopoly of health care, sanctioned by society, is now being challenged.

As we have seen, nurses as a predominantly female group, hold a subordinate position to medicine and the health bureaucracy. In turn, patriarchal oppression and inequitable power relations within the health care system impact on the way nurses relate to each other (Duffy, 1995). Examples of horizontal violence are common, where nurses, as relatively powerless members of the organisation, perpetuate overt and covert aggression towards each other. Criticism, undermining, scapegoating and infighting are common behaviours in nursing circles. It is no surprise that to avoid these behaviours from colleagues, nurses tend to be both conformist and compliant.

In addition, nurses have a caste system that values the thinkers (planners and prescribers) in nursing more than the doers (the implementers of care). As a result, the high-tech/less-touch practitioners (administration, education, coronary care, intensive care and accident and emergency)[4] are held in higher status than the low-tech/high-touch (medical, rehabilitation and geriatric nursing). Interestingly, it is within the non-acute medical environment where curing is not the central goal, that nurses have the opportunity to be on an equal level with other health care professionals.[5] Despite this, there is little evidence that nurses in the non-acute care sectors see themselves, or are viewed by others, as autonomous health professionals.

LEGAL ISSUES

A further structural barrier to the effective use of complementary health care is the relationship of nursing to the law. Previously, I discussed Menzies' thesis on nursing rituals as a defence against anxiety. She identified a rigid adherence to policies and procedures as one example of this process. Another reason given by nurses for their obsession with policies and procedures is the fear of litigation despite the fact that nurses are not sued very often.

The introduction of complementary therapies into nursing practice has generated a plethora of articles on the need to develop policies to ensure their safe implementation. Several nurses boards in Australia have responded to this cry by developing guidelines for the use of complementary therapies in nursing practice. The need to develop guidelines is curious, given that most complementary therapists claim that their therapies are safe in comparison with biomedical interventions, and that regulatory bodies have not responded in a similar fashion to the introduction of highly dangerous medical interventions that nurses must deliver.

Why is it that complementary therapies in nursing are seen to be potentially dangerous, and why are there not similar cries of concern and caution regarding the many and very dangerous medical interventions that we carry out? These concerns seem out of proportion to the real threat of adverse events, which currently occur on a daily basis, from drug interactions, polypharmacy, surgery, hospital acquired infections and medical negligence.

Complementary therapies are generally accepted as being safer and less invasive than allopathic medicine. Complementary nurse therapists who have a sound knowledge base in biomedicine as well as a complementary therapy are in an ideal position to deliver safe and effective care. Yet, Chiarella (1995:24), a nurse-lawyer, states that nurses need to exercise due care:

> *... which on occasions may mean that we have to be more conservative than non-nurse practitioners' (when working within the medical paradigm because) ... we cannot disregard one in favour of the other and still practice as an accredited nurse until these therapies are recognised by the public as things one could reasonably expect an accredited nurse to do.*
>
> (Chiarella, 1995:24).

Chiarella does not clarify her use of the term 'accredited'. The assumption is that she means a registered nurse who is also accredited in a complementary therapy. The suggestion that public recognition should be the arbiter of what an accredited nurse might reasonably practise is extraordinary, and yet another example of the view that nurses do not control their field of practice.

Megan-Jane Johnstone (1994:26), an Australian nurse ethicist, observes that:

> *The nursing legal literature … has been conspicuously silent on … the way the law operates in the specific field of nursing, and the role the law has played not only in obstructing the professional development of nursing, but also in supporting and maintaining nursing's continued subordination to the (male dominated) medical profession.*
>
> (Johnstone M-J 1994:26).

The nurses acts in Australia do not address therapeutic interventions. However, three nurses boards, whose primary role is the protection of the public[6], have developed guidelines for the use of complementary therapies in nursing practice. They give a broad overview of the issues involved, the central tenet being that nurses are responsible for their own safe, competent practice. The vexed issue as to whether a registered nurse who practises a complementary therapy is acting primarily in the capacity of nurse, complementary therapist or complementary nurse-therapist is not answered[7].

The Australian Nursing Council (ANCI, 1998) national competencies give no guidance about therapeutic interventions that may be regarded as reasonable for nurses to practise. In fact, many of the nursing competencies are so broad and general that they could apply to a range of therapists/professionals. Defining nursing practice is an impossible task and was abandoned by nurse theorists in the 1970s. Further, the development of professional standards for complementary therapies in nursing practice is difficult, given the broad range of therapies, their appropriateness to specific practice settings and whether they should be regarded as an integral part of nursing care or as complementary interventions. Nevertheless, expanding the scope of nursing practice is critical to the professional survival of nursing. Likewise, recognition of the right of nurses to incorporate complementary therapies into their practice must be addressed. Opponents of complementary therapies use the argument that there is the little scientific evidence of their effectiveness to limit practice in this field.

SCIENTIFIC PARADIGM

As complementary therapies are generally non-invasive and low risk in comparison to technological and pharmacological intervention, their introduction provides an ideal opportunity to incorporate holistic nursing care[8]. In particular, those therapies which require a high degree of physical and psychological contact, such as massage, aromatherapy and relaxation techniques, are appropriate to nursing practice. However, a profession may not value therapies because they lack 'scientific' status, for as O'Neill (1994a:124), points out in reference to acupuncture, modern science has become the patent for respectability.

Certainly, the concern about the lack of scientific evidence for some complementary therapies is justified. As yet there is not a substantial literature base[9] to confirm their effectiveness. However, there is an increasing body of research being undertaken by complementary nurse therapists and others that attest to their efficacy. Anecdotal evidence and the demand from the public for these therapies also suggests that many clients find them effective.

A further obstacle to the general acceptance of complementary therapies is the perceived mysticism that surrounds some of the therapies. Some proponents of energetic healing particularly, broach their discussion of healing with evangelistic fervour, leading the scientific rationalists to suspect that there is a connection between the therapy and some underlying religious belief. On the other hand, some Christian fundamentalists are concerned about the 'pagan' derivations of oriental healing philosophy and suspect 'new age' therapists of occult involvement and unChristian acts (Gennis, 1992).

Therapies that derive from alternative medical systems, such as traditional Chinese medicine and Ayurveda attract the greatest concern from scientific circles. There is apprehension about their potential to do harm as well as the lack of scientific validation of their effectiveness. Such concerns may be justified where two systems of medicine are used simultaneously. In particular, there may be hazards in using two therapies simultaneously, for example, herbal medicines may be contraindicated with particular pharmacological interventions. Likewise, some interventions are invasive and if used by incompetent or unskilled practitioners, they pose a threat of harm.

Until the establishment of the Office for Complementary Medicine in the Therapeutic Goods Administration (TGA) in 1999, there was no satisfactory regulation of complementary therapies in Australia and adverse events were not systematically monitored. It could be argued, however, that these therapies pose less of a threat than some current medical regimes.

PROFESSIONAL GATEKEEPING

Many of the arguments raised about 'safety' have more to do with professional gate keeping and control than a real threat to the patient's wellbeing. Whether a particular therapy is seen as harmless or potentially dangerous and in need of medical control is influenced by the stakeholders involved.

An interesting example is the attempt by medicine to control acupuncture. Until recently acupuncture was self-regulated and acupuncture courses of varying lengths and quality were offered by private providers[10]. Although acupuncture is based on an entirely different epistemology and system of medicine, medical practitioners were, until recently, able to practise acupuncture with a minimum of training (in some cases, a weekend workshop), the assumption being that their medical education provided an advanced level of knowledge. These inconsistencies, and the claim from several quarters that the therapies have the potential to do harm led to an inquiry into the regulation of acupuncture and traditional Chinese medicine in Victoria (Bensoussan and Myers, 1996). The intriguing contradiction here is that, although practitioners emphasise the safety of complementary therapies[11], their danger to the public when practised by unskilled practitioners was emphasised in the inquiry to convince the state that the industry should be regulated.

O'Neill (1994b:498) argues provocatively that:

> *If occupational practices were safe then that counted against practitioner registration. But if established medical groups said that alternative practitioners were dangerous and should be banned then that argument could be turned on its head; they could be made safe by regulation and the offer of appropriate education.*

Exclusive use of acupuncture is claimed on the grounds of safety. Until recently, in Victoria, registered nurses could undertake an 18-month diploma to become nurse-acupuncturists[12]. Following the establishment of a body to regulate traditional Chinese medicine, it is anticipated that the educational preparation of nurses and the use of the title acupuncturist by nurses will be reviewed. However, registered nurse-acupuncturists have won the right to choose whether to come under the jurisdiction of the Nurses Board of Victoria or the Chinese Medicine Registration Board, when it is established (RCNA, Connections 2000).

Another professional obstacle faced by complementary nurse-therapists is the limited remuneration provided by private insurers and public bodies such as Workcover and the Transport Accident Commission (TAC). Misconceptions about the provision of primary health care by nurses, in particular, diagnosis, treatment and referral, have led to anomalies in remuneration for their services. For example, a nurse who practises acupuncture cannot claim compensation from the TAC, whereas a physiotherapist or a chiropractor can. Issues surrounding primary contact practitioners will need to be resolved for complementary nurse practitioners to be economically viable.

A BLUEPRINT FOR CHANGE

Despite the popularity of complementary therapies and their appropriateness to nursing care, there are some major hurdles to overcome before they are accepted as an integral part of mainstream health care. There are many simple and effective therapies appropriate to nursing, for example, touch therapies including massage, relaxation therapies such as visual imagery, meditation and biofeedback, sound and music therapy, and using light and colour to create a healing environment. Nurses are also ideally situated to qualify and practise independently in a range of alternative therapies.

How can we reframe nursing care so that nurses have the courage and conviction to incorporate these therapies into their practice? The first step is to systematically address the forces that obstruct nurses from controlling their own practice. Promoting diversity and projecting professional confidence is one way in which to reframe the image of nursing practice. A deficient model of practice is currently portrayed, for example, in the Nurses Board of Victoria (1999) complementary therapy guidelines, phrases such as 'Nurses function within the limits of their education and competence and consult or refer . . .' give the clear perception of a clinician with limited education who is not in control of their practice. Consequently, nurses and other health professionals may view nurse complementary therapists as dabblers in an area that lacks credibility. The current debate and caution about the use of the term 'independent nurse practitioner' is another example of how nurses have unwittingly lost ground through an overly solicitous approach to autonomous practice.

Recognition and celebration of our skill, knowledge and expertise is essential if we are to raise the profile of nursing and claim professional ground. In nursing education, the inculcation of professional confidence, high self-esteem, and a sense of professionalism will assist in preparing graduates to take on a more independent role. Encouraging nurses to be creative and take risks is also an integral part of the process towards independent practice. A critique of educational and professional discourse to identify the perpetuation of a language of subordination and inferiority will assist in reframing a social system of repression. Maintaining professional and educational standards equal to those of other health professions is essential. Professional practice that is grounded in well documented empirical knowledge and research offers the opportunity to increase our credibility and raise the profile of nursing.

Altering the social and structural barriers within nursing is extremely hard because it requires changes in the system and behaviour change in nurses. Those of us who see the necessity to change the system (the reframing of health care to holistic health care) must work patiently and steadfastly to raise awareness, provide role models, educate, and support those with the courage to introduce innovative practice.

ENDNOTES

1. Some authors, for example, Bennett (1996) may dispute this.
2. I am referring here to nurses who are in paid employment.
3. The Quality in Australian Health Care Study (QAHS, 1996) estimated that adverse events (i.e. unintended injury) resulted in 3.3 million bed days per year, with a cost estimated at a tenth of all hospital expenditure.
4. In this environment, affectionate touch may be infrequent. See Clement (1983) and Schoenhofer (1989).
5. Davis and George (1998:232) suggest that an equal member team model is more likely in the non-acute setting than in acute care, where the emphasis is on curing and medicine dominates the health care team.
6. There is an erroneous belief in nursing circles that nurses boards have a responsibility to protect nurses.
7. The legal texts in nursing and complementary health care give no guidance on legal jurisprudence in dual professional roles and responsibilities.
8. Holistic care is a hallmark of most nursing curricula and many mission statements. At this stage, holistic care may be more rhetoric than reality.
9. The main exception to this is in the field of traditional Chinese medicine and acupuncture, which is now attracting funding from national research bodies such as the National Health & Medical Research Council.
10. The first undergraduate degree in acupuncture was offered in a Victorian university in 1992.
11. This claim may be justified, for, although there is no recent data, in 1982 a 12-month survey was conducted by the Victorian Health Commission and no adverse reactions to acupuncture were reported.
12. They may also undertake the other courses offered, however few of these give substantial credit towards existing knowledge gained through nursing. Subsequently, nurses may be required to do three to four years of training.

REFERENCES

Allan J, Hall B (1988): Challenging the focus on technology: A critique of the medical model in a changing health care system. *Advances in Nursing Science.* 10 (3):22-33.

Australian Nursing Council Inc, (1998): ANCI National Competency Standards for the Registered Nurse, 2nd edition. Canberra: ANCI.

Bennett J (1996): Holistic connections. *NSW Holistic Nurses Association Newsletter.* March: 3-4.

Besoussan A, Myers S, (1996): *Towards a safer choice: the practice of traditional Chinese medicine in Australia.* Campbelltown, NSW: Faculty of Health, University of West Sydney.

Bonawitt V, Evans M, (1994): *Legal and professional issues for nurses in Victoria in independent, private, or fee for service practice.* 6th Victorian state nursing, law and ethics conference, autonomy in nursing practice in the changing health care area: the ethical and legal responsibilities. RMIT, Melbourne.

Clement J (1983): *A descriptive study of the use of touch by nurses with patients in the critical care unit.* Doctoral thesis. Ann Arbor, UMI: University of Texas.

Chiarella M (1995) The magic of nursing: from witches and warriors to workers and wonders. *Australian Nursing Journal.* 3 (3): 22-24.

Dimond B (1998): *The Legal Aspects of Complementary Therapy Practice: a Guide for Health Care Professionals.* Sydney: Churchill Livingstone.

Duckett S (1984): Structural interests and Australian health policy. *Social Science and Medicine.* 18 (11): 959-966.

Duffy E, (1995): Horizontal violence: a conundrum for nursing. *Collegian.* 2 (2): 5-9, 12-17.

Gennis F, (1992): Alternative roads to Hell? *Nursing Standard* 6 (44): 42-43.

Grace H, (1990): Can Health Care Costs Be Contained? In: McLoskey J, Grace H, *Current Issues in Nursing.* St Louis: CV Mosby.

George J, Davis A (1998): *States of health: Health and illness in Australia.* South Melbourne: Longman.

Johnston M-J (1994): *Nursing and the Injustices of the Law.* Sydney: WB Saunders/Bailliere Tindall.

Jolley M, Brykczynska G (1993): *Nursing: Its Hidden Agendas.* Melbourne: Edward Arnold.

McCabe P (1994): Natural therapies in Australia: a nurse-naturopath's view. *Nurse Practitioner Forum.* 5 (2): 114-117.

McCabe P, Ramsay L, Taylor B (1995): *Complementary therapies in relation to nursing practice in Australia.* Discussion paper No. 2. Canberra: Royal College of Nursing Australia.

Menzies I (1970): *The Functioning of Social Systems as a Defence against Anxiety. A Report on a Study of the Nursing Service at a General Hospital.* London: The Tavistock Institute.

O'Neill A(1994a): *Enemies Within and Without.* Melbourne: La Trobe University Press.

O'Neill A (1994b): Danger and safety in medicines. *Social Science and Medicine.* 38 (4): 497-507.

Royal College of Nursing Australia (2000): Nurse acupuncturists and the registration of Chinese medicine. *RCNA Connections.* 3 (1): 21.

Schoenhoefer S, (1989): Affectional touch in critical care nursing: A descriptive study. *Heart & Lung.* 18 (2): 146-154.

Taskforce on Quality in Australian Health Care. *The Final Report of the Taskforce on Quality in Australian Health Care.* Canberra: Australian Government Publishing Service.

Taylor B (1997): Complementary therapies—fad or breakthrough? Paper presented at the conference 'Complementary therapies: increasing the experience of nursing' run by *Ausmed Publications*, Brisbane, 4-5 December, pp.1-9.

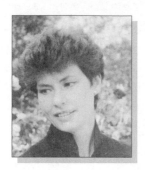

TRISHA DUNNING
PhD, RN, MEd, Grad Dip Ed (Health), Grad Dip Professional
Writing, Certificates in Obstetrics, Karitane, Family Planning,
Aromatherapy, Relaxation Massage, FRCNA

Clinical Nurse Consultant—Diabetes Education at St Vincent's
Hospital Melbourne

Trisha contributes to diabetes care through clinical practice, education and research, has published widely in the area, and is well known internationally as well as nationally. Combining complementary therapies and nursing was a natural step for Trisha. She acquired a love of herbs from her mother, a passion for the Australian bush from her dad, and learned holistic care from a local general practitioner in the NSW country town where she completed her nurse education. Trisha uses aromatherapy in her nursing practice and personal life. She is an active member of many committees, both in diabetes and complementary therapies. She is a member of the management committee of the Australian Complementary Health Association and in 1999 contributed regularly to *Nursing Review* about complementary therapies. Trisha lives on 17 acres with her animals, Australian plants, herb garden and husband.

Developing clinical practice guidelines

INTRODUCTION

The information presented in Chapters 2 and 3 indicates that half the Australian population uses some form of complementary therapy at some time. Therefore, it is no longer acceptable to ignore the use of complementary therapies in health care settings, particularly as many people bring their own therapies into hospital, or recommence them after they are discharged. It is appropriate then, to consider complementary therapies as part of the total assessment and management of individuals. The growing interest in and use of complementary therapies acknowledges the increasing evidence for the effect of an individual's psychological and emotional status on their physical wellbeing (Watkins, 1997). The widespread use of, and interest in, complementary therapies in the community is reflected in the increasing number of nurses and health professionals undertaking complementary therapy courses and using complementary therapies in patient care.

The integration of complementary therapies into nursing practice is a living process. In writing this chapter I would like to acknowledge those pioneer nurses committed to a holistic approach to care, who introduced complementary therapies into their practice, often without guidelines, and with potential medico-legal risks because of that lack.

In the past three years the nursing profession has recognised the need for guidelines to safeguard both patients and nurses, as well as to set common standards of complementary therapy care. A number of nursing organisations have issued guidelines for the use of complementary therapies, which can serve as a framework for the development of therapy specific and local guidelines, for example, the Nurses Boards of Victoria and Western Australia; Royal College of Nursing, Australia; Australian College of Holistic Nurses, and the Australian Nursing Federation. These beginnings indicate the growing importance of complementary therapies in nursing practice.

The work described in this chapter reflects the unique position I occupied in 1998 and 1999. During that period I convened a working party of the Nurses Board of Victoria (NBV) which reviewed the Board's *Guidelines for the Use of Complementary Therapies in Nursing Practice,* originally adopted in 1996. At the same time I chaired a working party at St Vincent's Hospital, Melbourne established to develop guidelines for the use of complementary therapies in the hospital.

The Board's Guidelines provide a professional context for using complementary therapies in nursing practice in terms of educational preparation, selection of therapies and professional considerations such as legislation, professional indemnity, informed consent and documentation. The Board's guidelines were designed to be used in conjunction with other relevant professional documents such as the Code of Professional Conduct for Nurses in Australia, Code of Practice for Midwives in Victoria, Code of Ethics and the Australian Nursing Council Competencies for the Registered and Enrolled Nurse. A comprehensive briefing paper was prepared to accompany the guidelines. It gives a comprehensive overview of issues relevant nurses with respect to complementary therapies in 1999.

WHY DEVELOP GUIDELINES?

One could ask if guidelines for the use of complementary therapies are necessary, since a number of complementary therapies are in fact nursing care. Likewise, many guidelines have been criticised for being narrow, reductionist, and not considering the consumer perspective. However, well constructed guidelines have many advantages and several reasons can be given for developing complementary therapies guidelines. They include, making provision for continuity of care across different health care sectors, limiting variation in health care practices and strengthening the link between research, evidence and clinical practice, thereby improving safety for patients and staff. In addition, guidelines are increasingly considered when standards of practice and benchmarks for care are being established.

From a practitioner's perspective guidelines can help clarify roles and responsibilities, enhance communication, define referral processes, and improve documentation.

Although guidelines have no status in law, they can be used as evidence of best or appropriate practice if such questions are considered by the courts or other investigative bodies. In this context guidelines are important to help identify and avoid foreseeable risks. A discussion of legal issues occurs in Chapter 5. Therefore, guidelines need to be broad enough to guide practitioners, without being unnecessarily prescriptive or inflexible. In the future, complementary therapies may well be a standard part of management and specific guidelines may no longer be necessary.

WHAT ARE GUIDELINES?

For the purpose of this discussion, 'guidelines' refers to systematically developed statements which assist the practitioner, and the patient, to make decisions about appropriate health care in specific circumstances (Institute of Medicine, 1992). They guide and complement clinical assessment and judgement, they do not replace it. The content detailed in specific practice guidelines is usually distilled from current evidence and/or the consensus opinion of experts about what constitutes best practice. Rarely, non-consensus guidelines are developed.

Guidelines are designated as either evidence based or consensus based, depending on the strength of the evidence that supports the statements made in the guidelines. Four broad levels of evidence are described:
• **Level i:** evidence derived from systematically reviewed randomised controlled trials
• **Level ii:** evidence derived from at least one randomised controlled trial
• **Level iii:** evidence derived from well described non-randomised controlled trials
• **Level iv:** evidence based on the opinion of respected, relevant authorities and derived from their experience, descriptive studies and reports of expert committees (United States Preventative Services Taskforce, 1989).

At this stage the evidence for most complementary therapies and complementary therapy guidelines falls into levels iii and iv. However, the amount of good quality research into complementary therapies is increasing, and a regular review process is desirable so that new research findings can inform the content of the guidelines and move them towards levels i and ii.

The presentation of guidelines takes many forms. Paper based formats are still the most frequently used but electronic guidelines are increasing in popularity. Guidelines may be more accessible if they are available in electronic formats.

CONSIDERATIONS FOR THE DEVELOPMENT OF GUIDELINES AT ST VINCENT'S

The need for guidelines for the use of complementary therapies in St Vincent's primarily grew out of the increasing number of patients bringing herbal and homeopathic remedies into the hospital and the widespread use of aromatherapy vapourisers. The use of complementary therapies was often an ad hoc process and clinical outcomes were not monitored. Therefore, guidelines were considered necessary to establish the parameters of safe practice and to ensure a consistent approach to the use of complementary therapies in the hospital.

In planning and developing the guidelines five main areas were considered, the educational preparation and competence of people practising complementary therapies, the safety and efficacy of various complementary therapy treatments, legal and ethical aspects of their use, ways to integrate complementary therapies into current management practices, and quality improvement and outcome monitoring processes. The fact that some practices appear to be bizarre, dangerous and untested was considered when determining which therapies would be appropriate for use in the hospital.

The Nurses Board of Victoria (NBV) *Guidelines for the Use of Complementary Therapies in Nursing Practice* (1999), (Appendix 3) were used as the overall framework in which to develop specific polices that would address the needs of St Vincent's Hospital. The guiding principles were that the guidelines needed to be:
• consistent with the mission and values of the hospital
• based on the best available evidence
• developed by a multidisclipinary team which included consumer representation
• complementary to orthodox care
• able to enhance the quality of care for individuals
• discussed with all relevant stakeholders
• flexible
• implemented, monitored and evaluated.

The aim was to identify specific processes that could ensure the best possible outcomes for patients and consider the effects of integrating complementary therapies into current nursing practice and patient care. In drafting the guidelines the working party sought to locate the best available evidence and to try to convert the evidence into clinically useful strategies to assist practitioners to incorporate complementary therapies into management plans and determine the suitability of complementary therapies for individual patients.

It is important to note that a wide variety of evidence was considered when developing the guidelines and was not restricted to randomised control trials. Considering a variety of levels of evidence was necessary because a great deal of the evidence for complementary therapies is derived from long traditional use and is contained in case reports and descriptive studies.

PROCESS FOLLOWED IN DEVELOPING THE GUIDELINES

The need for complementary therapy guidelines in the hospital was initially discussed with the chief nursing officer. Following these discussions, terms of reference and a strategic plan were developed. Once the content of these documents were agreed a working party was formed, and met regularly to review the literature and develop the guidelines.

The working party consisted of nurses with complementary therapy qualifications, a pharmacist, and a doctor. A consumer was consulted during the development of the guidelines but did not meet formally with the working party.

The purpose of the committee was to:
- develop policies and procedures for the use of complementary therapies in St Vincent's Hospital that conformed with safe ethical standards of practice and were evidence based where possible
- ensure the completed guidelines were consistent with the mission and values of the Sisters of Charity Health Service to which St Vincent's belongs
- determine which complementary therapies were appropriate to be used in the hospital based on the best available evidence for their safety and efficacy
- identify staff with particular qualifications and expertise in complementary therapies who could act as resource people for other staff.

A planned, stepwise developmental process was followed (see Table 3.1). The first step was to conduct a staff survey to ascertain how frequently complementary therapies were used in the hospital, staff knowledge about complementary therapies, the types of therapies in use, whether any staff had complementary therapy qualifications and to obtain an indication of the general feeling towards formally recognising the use of complementary therapies in the hospital. The survey questionnaire was anonymous and was distributed on the hospital e-mail network.

Table 3.1: Phases of guideline development utilised in the formulation of guidelines for St Vincent's Hospital

Phase	Activity
Phase 1	Need identified and discussed with Chief Nursing Officer.
	Staff survey to profile hospital use, identify resource people and flag the intention to develop complementary therapies guidelines.
Phase 2	Terms of reference and strategic plan developed. Working party formed.
Phase 3	Literature review and discussion with relevant experts and stakeholders. Draft document developed.
Phase 4	Staff invited to comment about the draft document. Comments analysed and incorporated into the document. Document submitted to hospital management committees.
*Phase 5	Implementation, integration, ongoing monitoring and evaluation.
*Phase 6	Review of literature and incorporation of new evidence into the guidelines.
* ongoing process.	

A small number of responses were received and all health professional groups were represented. A few had recognised complementary therapy qualifications and many, mostly nurses, reported an interest in complementary therapies. The survey also identified some staff concerns that complementary therapies was not appropriate for use in the hospital. Aromatherapy, massage of various types, music therapy, herbal medicine and homeopathy were the most frequently reported therapies in use at the time of the survey.

A process was already in place for ascertaining any actual or potential interactions between herbal, homeopathic and orthodox treatments. The process was designed to give patients and staff accurate information about using herbal products and orthodox treatments and at the same time to support their ability to make informed choices. This process became the basis for the use of these treatments in the final guidelines.

An extensive literature review was carried out and designated as 'the evidence'. The evidence was then given a rating according to the US Preventative Services Taskforce levels described earlier. Some existing guidelines for using complementary therapies in health care settings were identified but did not meet the needs of St Vincent's (Wafer, 1994; Fowler and Wall, 1997; and NSW Therapeutic Assessment Group Inc., 1999). Very little Level i or ii evidence was identified, which meant the guidelines would be predominantly consensus based.

CONTENT AREAS AND FORMAT OF THE GUIDELINES

The working party agreed that the complementary therapies already in use in the hospital and described above were appropriate as a starting point and guidelines were developed for these therapies initially. These therapy specific guidelines were set in a common framework that is applicable to all complementary therapies. In addition, a process whereby complementary therapies not covered in the guidelines could be considered if specifically requested was documented. The common framework sets out the background to the guidelines, gives the rationale for their development and defines the terms used in the guidelines as well as stating the aims and scope of the guidelines, the criteria for use of complementary therapies, the range of therapies the guidelines refer to and documentation and incident/adverse reaction reporting processes. The specific therapy guidelines describe aromatherapy, massage, and herbal medicine and homeopathy. The content of each of these guidelines addresses issues pertinent to the particular therapy. For example, the aromatherapy guidelines include information about the selection, labelling and storage of essential oils.

Once the draft guidelines were completed the hospital staff were informed that they were available for comment via the hospital e-mail system. The draft document was sent to individuals for comment when requested. Feedback and comments were received from a range of health professionals and were for the most part positive and constructive in nature. Where appropriate the suggestions were integrated into the document. The major headings used in the common, and specific guidelines are shown in Table 3.3.

Table 3.2:   Factors influencing the success of clinical management guidelines

Factors influencing success	Factors which may inhibit use of guidelines
Consultation with relevant stakeholders	Prescriptive and inflexible
Flexible, logical, consistent and readily accessible at the point of care	Outside the level of competence and knowledge of staff
Act as a checklist to guide clinical care planning	The belief that the guidelines will be used to take the place of individual clinical assessment and judgement
Relevant to the needs of staff and patients	Limited access to the document and complex information
Accompanied by education and ongoing monitoring	A belief that the guidelines have been over-simplified, or fail to address the complexity of practice and key issues.

IMPLEMENTATION AND INTEGRATION INTO PRACTICE

The completed guidelines were ratified through the Hospital's management and senior staff committees. Recommendations about a suitable integration process were made when the completed document was presented to management. The recommendations addressed the following core elements of integration:

- education about the guidelines and the reasons for using complementary therapies in the hospital so that staff gain an understanding of the principles of holism and see complementary therapies as a normal part of care
- outcome monitoring, including adverse events
- respect for the patient's right to make informed choices
- multidisciplinary co-operation
- evaluation and revision of the guidelines.

As well as addressing these core elements the optimal integration of guidelines into practice depends on organisational factors, available resources and defined processes for delivery. These issues will be the responsibility of individual clinical areas where complementary therapies are used. In effect, integration involves bridging the gap between current practice and desired practice and requires time, patience, respect and open communication. A number of factors affect the success of clinical management guidelines and these are shown in Table 3.2.

Table 3.3:   Major headings used in the St Vincent's Hospital common and specific guidelines

Common guidelines	Aromatherapy	Herbal medicines and homeopathy	Massage
Introduction	Introduction	Introduction covering legislation, approval and regulation of herbal remedies	Introduction
Rationale	Definition of terms	Definition of terms	Definitions
Scope of the guidelines	Essential oils and application methods	Criteria for use	Contraindications and precautions
Aims	Storage	Consent and documentation	Massage and essential oils
Criteria for use	Consent and documentation	Supply of herbal products	Consent and documentation
Range of therapies to be used	Reporting adverse reactions	Administration	References
Consent	Disposal of unused oils	Storage	
Accountability and competence	References	Disposal of unused products	
Documentation		Reporting adverse reactions	
Definition of terms		References	

As with any change in practice, a process whereby the implementation and outcomes of the guidelines can be overseen and monitored is vital. The working party recommended that a standing committee be appointed to address these issues. The guidelines will be incorporated into the Hospital Policy Manual. Thus they will be linked to and consistent with existing processes such as documentation, outcome monitoring and adverse drug reaction reporting, which will enhance their acceptance and usefulness. Incorporating the complementary therapy guidelines and orthodox care guidelines in one manual enhances the likelihood that complementary therapies will be seen as part of a holistic approach to care, rather than as separate and different.

There is some evidence that guidelines that operate within the practitioner/patient consultation and focus on individual patients are more likely to lead to changes in practice (Grimshaw and Russell, 1993). It is expected that nurses with expertise in complementary therapies will utilise therapies in the care of individual patients. Thus, this parameter will be operating as our guidelines are implemented. In reality, the integration and wide acceptance of the guidelines will depend to a large extent on local human resource issues, job descriptions, finances and lines of clinical decision making. Each clinical area of the hospital is responsible for its own budget, rosters and work allocation. Complementary therapies will be considered along with other relevant planning issues. It was difficult to give any cost-benefit information for complementary therapies that could assist with budget planning as only limited economic appraisals exist.

It is expected that complementary therapies will be incorporated into patient care in a variety of ways and at different levels depending on staff knowledge and competence as defined in the Nurses Board of Victoria guidelines (NBV, 1999). The NBV guidelines describe the level at which complementary therapies may be used by nurses according to their knowledge and competence and provides a framework that assists nurses to make decisions about their role with respect to complementary therapies, and the level at which they should practise. A thorough nursing assessment is the basis for determining if a complementary therapy is appropriate for individual patients and should be undertaken before a complementary therapy is prescribed.

DIFFICULTIES ENCOUNTERED

There were few difficulties encountered in meeting the terms of reference and strategic plan deadlines, but there were some unavoidable delays in the adoption and promulgation of the guidelines. A few staff members, primarily medical staff, expressed concerns that the standing of the hospital would be compromised if 'unscientific' practices were condoned for use in the hospital. These concerns were respected and acknowledged. The reasons for developing guidelines were discussed with the staff concerned and they were invited to comment about the guidelines. By adopting a conciliatory approach a major confrontation and possible rejection of the guidelines was avoided.

MEASURING THE SUCCESS OF THE GUIDELINES

The successful implementation of the guidelines will depend on their sensitivity to the needs of the staff members working with the guidelines, the accessibility of the guidelines in terms of the language used and the overall design of the document as well as where it is located in the clinical areas. These issues will be monitored under existing hospital quality management processes.

The evaluation will be divided into short-term and long-term evaluation. Short-term evaluation will address change in current practice (for example use of electric vapourisers instead of candle heated vapourisers) and changes in staff knowledge and attitudes about complementary therapies. In the longer term changes in the way complementary therapies are viewed and improved health outcomes for patients will be measured. It is also a personal hope that the guidelines will encourage good quality research into complementary therapies and improved documentation of their use and the outcomes achieved.

Specific clinical outcome indicators will be monitored based on the reason for using each complementary therapy. Most of this data will be collected for individual patients and may include relief of symptoms such as pain, nausea, sleeplessness and mood. Routine outcomes to be monitored include, the frequency with which the guidelines are used, patient and staff satisfaction with the guidelines and the specific therapy, and the frequency of incidents/adverse reactions. These parameters are the same as those monitored for orthodox care. Importantly, a time frame for revising the guidelines and incorporating new evidence into the guidelines was set.

REFERENCES

Australian Nursing Council (ANCI) (1998): *National Competency Standards for the Registered and Enrolled Nurse*. Canberra: ANC.

Australian Nursing Council (ANCI), (1993): *Code of Ethics for Nurses in Australia*. Canberra: ANCI.

Australian Nursing Council (ANCI) (1995): *Code of Professional Conduct for Nurses in Australia*. Canberra: ANCI.

Nurses Board of Victoria (NBV) (1999): *Code of Practice for Midwives in Victoria*. Melbourne: NBV.

Australian Nursing Federation (ANF)—Federal Office (1996): *Policy Statement: Complementary and Alternative Therapies*. Canberra: ANF.

Fowler P, Wall M (1997): COSHH and CHIPS: Ensuring the safety of aromatherapy. *Complementary Therapies in Medicine*. (5): 112-115.

Grimshaw J, Russell I (1993): Effect of clinical guidelines on medical practice: a systematic review of rigorous evaluations. *The Lancet*. 342: 1317-1322.

Institute of Medicine (1992): *Guidelines for Clinical Practice: from development to use*. Field M, Lohr K (eds). Washington DC: National Academy Press.

National Health and Medical Research Council (1995): *Guidelines for the Development and Implementation of Clinical Practice Guidelines*. Canberra: AGPS.

NSW Therapeutic Assessment Group Inc. (1999): Complementary Medicines in public hospitals, a discussion paper. Sydney: NSW Health Department.

Nurses Board of Victoria (1999): *Guidelines for the Use of Complementary Therapies in Nursing Practice*. Melbourne.

Nurses Board of Western Australia (1996): *Guidelines for the Use of Complementary Therapies in Nursing*. Perth.

Royal College of Nursing Australia, Position Statement: *Complementary Therapies in Australian Nursing Practice*. Canberra.

US Preventative Services Taskforce Report (1989): *Guide to Clinical Preventative Services: an Assessment of the Effectiveness of 169 Interventions*. M Fisher (ed.) Maryland. Williams and Wilkins.

Wafer M (1994): Finding the formula to enhance care. Guidelines for the use of complementary therapies in nursing practice. *Professional Nurse* March: 414-417.

Watkins A (1997): *Mind Body Medicine*. New York: Churchill Livingstone.

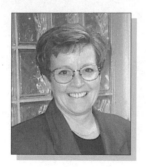

ELAINE DUFFY
RN, Midwife, Tropical Diseases Dip (London), Dip App Science (Community Health Nursing), Maternal & Child Health Cert, B App Sci (Advanced Nursing) (Lincoln Institute, Melbourne), Master of Nursing (Education major) (PIT, Melbourne), Therapeutic Touch Level 1 Certificate, FRCNA

Associate Professor and Associate Director at the Monash University Centre for Rural Health, Latrobe Regional Hospital, Traralgon, Victoria

Elaine has been teaching for 13 years, 11 of which have been in the higher education sector. She was a founding member of the Caroline Chisholm School of Nursing at Frankston where nursing programs commenced in 1987. In her current position at the Centre for Rural Health, Elaine is involved in research, teaching, supervision and projects. She teaches several subjects by distance education in the Graduate Diploma/Master of Rural Health course, including Aboriginal health and complementary health care. She is a beginning practitioner in therapeutic touch.

Elaine emigrated to Australia from England in 1976. She went to Darwin where she worked in Aboriginal health in remote Northern Territory and learned a great deal about herself and about indigenous culture. In 1982, Elaine settled in Melbourne and worked in community health, moving into the higher education sector in 1986. Elaine completed a Masters Degree in Nursing in 1991, and is currently undertaking a PhD at Monash University. She lives on a 10-acre property in rural Glengarry, surrounded by natural bush and native flora and fauna.

Chapter 4

Education and professional development

INTRODUCTION

Complementary therapies have gained significant recognition and credibility in recent years. According to Lloyd et al. (1993) changes in social and cultural attitudes and beliefs about allopathic medicine coincided with a growth in the popularity of complementary therapies. People are disenchanted with allopathic medicine and a better educated and more discriminating public is disillusioned with experts in general and sceptical about science and positivist knowledge. At the same time, health professionals, particularly nurses and midwives, express disillusionment with the health system, which they describe as impersonal and mechanistic, a system that relies heavily on costly technologies and drugs many with potent side effects.

In the modern health care system, cure as repair of the body is commonplace. Advancements in biomedical technology give doctors a wider variety of spare parts to replace diseased organs, blood vessels and other body parts (Gerber, 1988). The onset of illness, especially if severe, constitutes a threat to the integrity of the whole person. In the modern 'sick' care context, the person often becomes dehumanised in order for healing, or more commonly, for curing to occur. The person becomes fragmented, reduced to concrete parts, disembodied, objectified, and physically defined in time and space, for the treatment, removal, or manipulation of some part of the body or mind.

The recognition of 'complementary' therapies as an integral part of the health care system has developed rapidly and continues to gain momentum, despite the negative connotations and attitudes of some orthodox health professionals. A significant achievement at the end of the twentieth century for example, is the attainment of degree accreditation for courses in naturopathy. This chapter outlines a brief history of healing and the role of women and explores the advancements of undergraduate and postgraduate nursing education and other professional developments in the field of complementary therapies.

Complementary therapies have been variously described as 'alternative', 'unorthodox', 'marginal', 'fringe' and 'quackery'. These labels marginalise therapies other than orthodox medicine. In a sociological analysis of complementary healers, Willis (1994) describes the contradictory position of complementary therapies in contemporary society and in the context of medical dominance. At one level, he argues, complementary therapies continue to blossom in the face of opposition and hostility from the medical profession, and at another level, the efficacy of the therapeutic techniques of these complementary therapies remains questionable according to the canons of scientific evidence.

Despite continued opposition and hostility from orthodox practitioners, and the putative claims of unsubstantiated 'scientific' research, interest in and demand for complementary therapies continue to expand at an exponential rate. According to Charles Fogliani (cited in Spencer, 1998), 'half the Australian population visited practitioners in the $1 billion industry' of complementary therapies. This indicates a high level of interest in complementary therapies and a high degree of acceptance by the public.

The term 'complement' refers to wholeness, completeness, and integrality. These terms are all too familiar in the 'modern' health/sick care system, but in practice, often echo rhetoric rather than reality. The roots of the words 'heal' and 'health' are derived from the Anglo-Saxon word **haelan**, which means to be or to become whole (Quinn, 1984). For Dossey et al. (1995), holism involves studying and understanding the interrelationships of the bio-psycho-social-spiritual dimensions of the person, recognising that the whole is greater than the sum of its parts. The individual is seen as a dynamic integrated whole, interacting with, and being acted upon by their internal and external environments.

Healing and health espouse the harmony of mind–body–spirit (Quinn, 1984; and Watson, 1985) and thus the wholeness and integrity of the person. The next section gives a brief overview of the history of healing and the gendered nature of healing, outlining the subversion of female healers and healing knowledge.

HISTORY OF HEALING: BRIEF OVERVIEW

Throughout history, in many societies, the origin of illness and the process of healing have been related to spiritual sources. Notions of wholeness, balance and harmony with the universe were, and continue to be, central concepts of ancient healing and holistic philosophies. For much of history women were the healers. The Greek goddesses Hygeia and Panacea represented healing and prevention and their mother Epione was the patron saint of those in pain.

The Greek traditions formed what was considered to be the epitome of healing practices in Western civilisation until about four hundred years ago. Some scholars believe that the female healers of ancient Greece (2000 BC) were largely responsible for the initial development of surgical techniques and therapeutics, which made Greek medicine the most advanced in the ancient world (Achterberg, 1990).

Women healers owned a snake entwined staff, or caduceus, for the purpose of healing. Today the snake entwined staff is symbolic of medicine. It is interesting that Greek women healers were pictured in art form as keepers of the snake. The snake is the symbol of feminine healing energy (Achterberg, 1990). It is ironic that the caduceus, an ancient female symbol, now represents modern medicine, and reference is made to the 'founding fathers' of medicine, Aristotle, born in the third century BC and Hippocrates, born 460 BC.

Pythias, the wife of Aristotle, whom he referred to as his 'assistant', carried out research into tissues and reproduction using chicken and human embryos. It is probable that women like Pythias contributed significantly to the research and writings of 'modern medicine', however, there is little documentation to support this contention. Jeanne Achterberg (1990) suggests that the prolific writings of Aristotle, Hippocrates and Galen consisted of the research and works of many writers, including women, who were never acknowledged.

Women's legitimate right to practise healing was gradually eroded by changing societal mores and religious dogma. The role of women as healers, with intuitive insights, was brought to an end with the emergence of religious institutions dominated by men. By the Middle Ages, female healers and midwives were burned at the stake because it was believed they were witches, acting on behalf of the devil.

Throughout the Middle Ages, women's involvement in healing and their contribution to the creation of knowledge in medicine and science was often discarded, plagiarised and/or not acknowledged (Achterberg, 1990; and Stein, 1990). Women were excluded from education programs and indeed from possessing knowledge, unless it was sanctioned by men Thus, the processes of the masculinisation and medicalisation of healing practices and knowledge had begun and continues today to a lesser degree. In contemporary society, women in the community, in practice and in academia, are now creating counter discourses that challenge the dominant medical discourses on health, illness and healing knowledge.

Since the latter half of the nineteenth century, Western medical science, based on the world views of Rene Descartes and Isaac Newton, has dominated medical and nursing education and practice. This mechanistic viewpoint sees the person as a collection of concrete parts and chemicals; the mind and body functioning independently; and processes and events occurring in a predictable way, according to rigid laws and principles. The theories of mechanistic science are being challenged, particularly with developments in quantum physics, which conceptualises the human body and the universe as a unified network of energy.

A medical practitioner, Gerber (1988), describes this phenomenon as the 'Einsteinian' paradigm, in which human beings are seen as networks of complex energy fields, that interface with physical/cellular systems. He suggests that specialised forms of energy healing can be used to positively affect those energetic systems, that may be out of balance due to disease states. This view forms the basis of therapies such as reiki, therapeutic touch and kinesiology.

Nurses and midwives are challenging generations of indoctrination with the mechanistic world view, which has impacted on how they practise. There is widespread dissatisfaction amongst nurses and midwives, and society is becoming disenchanted with orthodox medical and nursing practices (Pfiel, 1994; Thurtle, 1993; and Trevelyan, 1993). Holistic nursing and midwifery, with the inclusion of complementary therapies, offers new visions for practice and health care.

NURSING AND MIDWIFERY: NEW VISIONS

Reid (1994) argues that nursing and midwifery have retained the 'old' skills of the female healers of the past. The use of complementary therapies in these disciplines is associated with caring for the whole person, in partnership, giving quality time and attention, and using intuitive skills (Wright, 1995). Helen Passant, a clinical nurse specialist in complementary therapies in the United Kingdom, describes how touch and massage changed the lives of not only the elderly patients in her care, but also the lives of the nurses providing therapy (Passant, 1991). The use of complementary therapies as an adjunct to holistic nursing practice could not only lead to improvements in patient care but also could provide a more satisfying and fulfilling role for the nurse and midwife (Armstrong and Waldron, 1991).

According to Teschendorff and Chew (1993), nurses are increasingly seeing themselves as facilitators of the healing process, taking an active rather than a passive role. This is a new vision for nurses, who have adopted a passive and secondary role to orthodox medicine in the past. For Rankin-Box (1993), the use of complementary therapies in nursing practice could be seen as a sign of the developing status of nursing and midwifery as disciplines, in which nurses and midwives are still clarifying the parameters of their professional activities.

The ever increasing community dissatisfaction with health care and technology and the demand for other forms of care, coupled with nurses' and midwives' disillusionment with technologically driven practice, combine to re-create a broader conceptualisation of nursing practice that incorporates complementary therapies. Nurses, midwives and other health professionals must support the promotion and acceptance of complementary therapies if the therapies are to be accepted as integral components of care (Pfiel, 1994; and Rankin-Box, 1993).

Stevenson (1992) and Tiran (1992) caution nurses and midwives not to 'dabble' in therapies about which they have inadequate knowledge and experience. Some practitioners complete short courses and then believe they are qualified to practise the therapy and teach it to others. Education and accountability are therefore, very important.

The introduction of complementary therapies in both the practice and education domains should be treated with caution, because some people view such ideas with suspicion and scepticism. In a survey of nurses by Arndt et al. (1995) in Victoria, Australia, participants were asked: 'What difficulties have you encountered or might you encounter as constraints to introducing complementary therapies in your nursing practice?' Responses referred to the closed minds of colleagues, insular attitudes of peers, lack of knowledge and understanding, and comments that included 'non-scientific' and 'lack of research', as well as 'quackery' and a 'waste of time'. Arndt's findings are significant as they highlight the suspicious and often sceptical views held by nurses in the practice domain.

However, in the same survey, a group of post registration Bachelor of Nursing (BN) students was asked if they used complementary therapies in their practice. Of the 47 responses obtained, 42 (87%), indicated they used complementary therapies in nursing practice. A range of therapies were identified including acupuncture, aromatherapy, crystals, massage, religious icons, music, relaxation, stress management and vitamin and mineral therapy (Arndt, 1995). This finding was significant, highlighting major implications for education.

The acceptance and use of complementary therapies in nursing practice and education for practice is critical (Booth, 1993; and Rankin-Box, 1993). The potential for complementary therapies to be discredited lies with nurses and other health practitioners who claim practice rights and expertise in a therapy, but have insufficient preparation. However, nurses and professional nursing organisations in Australia and overseas recognise the need to develop nursing and education policies that address standards of practice, competence and appropriate education requirements.

PROFESSIONAL DEVELOPMENT

Since 1993, several major initiatives have occurred in Australia with respect to introducing complementary therapies into nursing practice and education. In 1996, for example, the Australian Nursing Federation (ANF) Federal Council, adopted a policy statement titled *Complementary and Alternative Therapies* (see Appendix 1). The document identifies the complex nature of complementary therapies that influences the type of education required to practise safely and effectively. Further, the document points to the importance of seeking accredited education programs particularly for highly specialised modalities and those which can cause harm such as acupuncture and aromatherapy.

In 1995, the Royal College of Nursing, Australia (RCNA), the national professional body for nurses, produced a discussion document titled *Complementary Therapies in Relation to Nursing Practice in Australia* (McCabe et al., 1994). Subsequently, a position statement, *Complementary Therapies in Australian Nursing Practice,* was developed and published in 1997 (see Appendix 2). These position statements highlight the importance of employer policies, and the development of guidelines for the use of complementary therapies in health facilities.

These documents focus on major issues that require debate amongst nurses. These issues include the implications of using complementary therapies in practice and education and research, as well as raising relevant political considerations. Further, in 1995, the Nurses Board of Victoria (NBV) established a working party whose brief was to explore the development of nursing policy, standards, education and competencies for the inclusion of complementary therapies in nursing practice. *Guidelines for Use of Complementary Therapies in Nursing Practice* were produced by the Nurses Board of Victoria (NBV) in 1995 and revised in 1999 (NBV, 1999) (see Appendix 3). The NBV guidelines outline education, practice, referral and professional considerations.

For reasons of safety, the nursing and midwifery professions must identify those therapies that can be safely and effectively introduced, and determine the minimum education requirements necessary to include complementary therapies in nursing practice (Gates, 1993).

The addition of complementary therapies to nursing practice in Australia is guided, to a large degree, by the general statement for nurses undertaking clinical practice/procedures outlined in state nurses acts. The following extracts from the *Victorian Nurses Act* (1993) could encompass the use of complementary therapies, provided nurses can demonstrate adequate preparation and competence to practice.

> *Each nurse is accountable for his/her practice ... accordingly, nurses should carry out only those clinical procedures for which they have been prepared ... this should include theory and supervised practice until the nurse has been assessed as competent.*

> **and**

> *Nurses are at all times responsible for their own acts. They are expected to be aware of the limits of their abilities and to function within these limits.*
>
> *(Victorian Nurses Act, 1993).*

The NBV policy document reiterates the need for nurses to function within the limits of their education and competence in relation to complementary therapies as they do in other areas of practice. These extracts make explicit the necessity for adequate educational preparation for competent practice. It is difficult to determine what constitutes adequate educational preparation. A continuing cause for concern is the plethora of courses offered in different therapies through a variety of formal and informal programs. The content and length of courses differ. Some courses offer in-depth conceptual foundations of a particular therapy, while others provide short programs, workshops, and seminars. A guide developed by the Royal College of Nursing, United Kingdom, and adapted by McCabe (1999) for the Australian context, identifies some of the factors to consider when choosing a complementary therapy course (see Appendix 4.1 at the end of Chapter 4).

According to Willis (1994), these variations are reflective of differences in philosophy and preferred treatments of the various complementary therapies. More importantly, he argues, the variety of therapies may be seen as occurring along a continuum of 'legitimacy', with chiropractic, osteopathy, naturopathy and traditional Chinese medicine at one end, shading off into more esoteric and spiritual modalities at the opposite end of the spectrum. Further, some therapies, such as chiropractic and acupuncture, require more in-depth study for the purpose of registration to practise. Others, such as therapeutic touch (TT), require certification, because registration is not yet required. In these cases it is interesting to note that the relevant professional body, the TT Society, has developed a code of practice to describe safe practice. In 1998, the Victorian parliament accepted the 1996 recommendation of Bensoussan and Myers to provide statutory registration for traditional Chinese practitioners (Jacka, 1998).

According to Willis (1994) the degree of legitimacy of various complementary therapies rests on three important principles: first, how practitioners are educated into a paradigm of knowledge; second, the attainment of a recognised degree as the basis for registration; and third, certification that the individual has the knowledge and competence to practice. Chiropractic and osteopathy have achieved legitimacy on the grounds that the educational preparation, now in the higher education sector, achieves these criteria.

Further, the practice of chiropractic has been contained within a discourse of safety that places boundaries around the extent of practice. The safest ground and most secure occupational territory is in the treatment of musculoskeletal (Type 'M') problems, such as back problems. Practice within legal parameters, therefore, relies on compliance with this limited practice and will be enhanced by de-emphasising its ability to treat organic or visceral conditions (Willis, 1994).

EDUCATION: NEW VISIONS

Curricula and awards available at various universities and colleges are not yet standardised so individual institutions design curricula and decide the type of award they will offer (McCabe et al., 1995). The debate about the content of curricula in complementary therapies is whether medical science should form the basis of these courses and if so to what degree. The arguments for the inclusion of medical science in curricula, is based on the concept of 'legitimacy' and the dominant discourses of medical scientific knowledge. The argument was summed up by O'Neill (1994:106), who stated that entrenched beliefs about the putative 'truth-equals-science' type were uppermost whenever 'registration' or higher education courses in complementary therapies were blocked.

Further, Rankin-Box (1995) highlights the variation in entry requirements, some institutions being stringent while others make assumptions about the knowledge levels and competency of students, particularly when they have qualifications in a health related course. The allocation of credit for existing qualifications adds another dimension to the education debate. Medical practitioners and their putative claims to authoritative scientific knowledge in their basic degree, appear to obtain the most credit towards courses in complementary therapies, such as acupuncture. This is ironic in that medical education focused on a scientific or 'Newtonian' paradigm rather than a holistic 'Einsteinian' paradigm until very recently.

In the past, nursing education was influenced by the dominance of a narrow biomedical paradigm, which emphasised medical technology, mechanistic care, and bionic developments. The counter discourse of holism, based on the premise that the human person is more than the sum of individual parts, is seen to be more congruent with nursing care and nursing practice. As nursing encompasses a holistic paradigm to guide practice, nursing education programs will need to reflect the changed philosophical standpoint.

Nursing faculties in Australia are beginning to explore the possibilities of undergraduate and postgraduate education in appropriate natural therapies, such as, therapeutic touch, massage and meditation, which appears to be a strategy to resist medical dominance and to focus more on primary care (Jacka, 1998).

UNDERGRADUATE EDUCATION

In some universities, where discipline-specific complementary therapy courses have not yet been achieved, complementary therapies are introduced in undergraduate nursing degree courses as compulsory or elective units of study, the aim being to broaden the students' concept of complementary therapies, their benefits in the healing process and appropriate application of these therapies in nursing practice. In this way, students develop a beginning knowledge of the subjects covered, an open minded approach to both conventional and complementary healing practices and a changed focus from high technology care to facilitation of the patient's participation in the healing process (Teschendorff and Chew,1993; and Milton and Lewis,1993).

In 1995 the Southern Cross University in New South Wales implemented a full time three year Bachelor of Health Sciences (Naturopathy) program offered through the Centre for Nursing and Health Care Practices (Jacka, 1998; and Ramsay,1994). Since that time a separate School of Naturopathy has been established and offers undergraduate programs.

An elective unit titled *Introduction to Natural Therapies* for the Bachelor of Health Sciences, Nursing, course was developed at the Southern Cross University in Lismore, NSW (Jacka, 1998). This elective was the third most popular unit with distance education nursing students according to McCabe et al. (1995). Other universities are offering undergraduate degrees in specific complementary therapy modalities and provide bridging courses for individuals who have degrees in medicine, nursing, physiotherapy and occupational therapy. At RMIT University, for example, the Faculty of Biomedical and Health Sciences and Nursing is offering a Bachelor Degree program in Chinese medicine, which includes acupuncture, from the year 2000. In the second year of the two year full time degree a clinical internship will be offered in China. A double degree in nursing and naturopathy designed by the School of Nursing at LaTrobe University in Victoria will be available in 2001.

POSTGRADUATE EDUCATION

A Master of Applied Science (Acupuncture) will commence during the year 2000 at RMIT and will be open to primary health professionals with a relevant degree. It is a three year part time course that incorporates a graduate certificate after year one, a graduate diploma after year two and a master's degree after three years.

MULTIDISCIPLINE EDUCATION

Rankin-Box (1995) argues that it would be misleading to think that complementary therapies are part of a continuum of nursing practice. She advocates a multidiscipline approach to training in complementary therapies, which would challenge the emergence of distinct programs oriented towards any single health professional group. Rankin-Box's argument is based on the premise that multidiscipline education could serve to ensure therapeutic competence regardless of the background of practitioners. She argues that the emergence of complementary therapies in health care today should represent a 'muddling of vocational identities', whereby there is an intention to construct synthesised roles and education programs, and to group students together to develop competent and knowledgeable practitioners of integrated healing in clinical practice.

The call for multidiscipline education in complementary therapies is philosophically sound and appears appropriate in the current context of health professional education. However, the political implications of this notion are far reaching. For example, at present there is a monopoly of control over health care, the education of health professionals, and the legitimation of knowledge and practice. A challenge to the status quo of health care inevitably involves politics.

As complementary therapies move into the higher education sector, they are gradually being introduced into nursing courses as modalities of care and holistic nursing. The underlying philosophies of complementary therapies and nursing practice have a common and central aim, that of facilitating healing within a holistic framework.

As part of the multidiscipline Graduate Diploma/Master of Rural Health, offered by the Monash University Centre for Rural Health, a new subject, Complementary Therapies in Rural Practice, was developed and is offered by distance education (Duffy et al., 1997). It provides an introduction to complementary therapies for rural health practitioners. Similarly, the School of Health at the University of New England offers a unit of study by distance education as part of its open campus program for practitioners from various disciplines. The unit, Complementary Therapies in the Health Care System, focuses on a critical analysis of biomedicine and complementary therapies from a broad social, economic, historical and political context. These developments in education are testament to the growing recognition of complementary therapies as credible, academic pursuits in the health professional community and in the political context.

CONCLUSION

The vision of an Australian health care system, where current conventional health care practice is enhanced by the integration of a variety of complementary healing therapies, to provide genuine holistic care for the client/patient community, is a vision shared by many Australian nurses. An awareness of different world views and belief systems amongst those responsible for developing nursing and health curricula could lead to the incorporation of the philosophies of East and West, thereby enhancing nurse education. The inclusion of complementary therapies into nursing programs will enable a reconceptualisation of nursing roles, in particular, the role of active facilitator in the healing process.

In conclusion, we have much to learn from the healers of the past, whose wisdom and foresight have been subsumed into contemporary medicalised health. However, a renaissance of the underlying beliefs and philosophies of the 'old realities' of ancient times has created 'new visions'. These visions in turn have stimulated a reconceptualisation of humanity, healing, nursing and education. For these new visions to be realised, ancient healing knowledge needs to be incorporated into the development of health professional curricula and integrated into clinical care. In this way we can achieve the profound goal of holistic nursing within a holistic health care system.

REFERENCES

Achterberg J (1990): *Woman as healer: A panoramic survey of the healing activities of women from prehistoric times to the present.* Boston: USA: Shambhala. Publications Inc.

Armstrong F, Waldron R (1991): A complementary strategy. *Nursing Times.* 87 (11): 34-35.

Arndt C, Brown F, Johnstone J, Knight M, Medhurst A (1995): *Complementary therapies in nursing practice.* Paper presented to Professional Issues in Nursing conference: Frankston, Monash University.

Australian Nursing Federation (1996): Policy Statement: *Complementary and Alternative Therapies.* Melbourne: ANF.

Booth B (1993): Healthy alternatives? Complementary therapies. *Nursing Times.* 89 (17): 34-36

Byrne C (1992): Research methods in complementary therapies. *Nursing Standard.* 6 (50): 54-56.

Dossey B, Keegan L, Guzzetta CE, Kolkmeier LG (1995*): Holistic Nursing: a Handbook for Practice* (2nd ed). Maryland: Aspen Publishers Inc.

Gates B (1994): The use of complementary and alternative therapies in health care: a selective review of the literature and discussion of the implications for nurse practitioners and health care managers. *Journal of Clinical Nursing.* 3 (1): 43-47.

Gerber R (1996): *Vibrational Medicine: New Choices for Healing Ourselves* (2nd ed). Santa Fe, New Mexico: Bear & Company.

Jacka J (1998): *Natural Therapies: the Politics and Passion.* Ringwood: Ringwood Natural Therapies Inc.

Lloyd P, Lupton D, Wiesner D, Hasleton S (1993): Choosing alternative therapy: an exploratory study of sociodemographic characteristics and motives of patients resident in Sydney. *Australian Journal of Public Health.* 17 (2): 135-144.

Milton G, Lewis J (1993): Old links and new connections: traditional medicine and complementary healing modalities. London, UK, Teaching women's health: A multidisclipinary conference for teachers of medicine and nursing.

McCabe P, Ramsay L, Taylor B (1995): *Complementary Therapies in Relation to Nursing in Australia.* Canberra: RCNA.

Nurses Act (1993) No. 111/193 Victoria: Australia.

Nurses Board of Victoria (1999): *Guidelines for the Use of Complementary Therapies in Nursing Practice.* Melbourne: Australia, NBV.

O'Neill A (1994): *Enemies Within and Without.* Melbourne, Australia: Latrobe University Press.

Passant H (1991): A renaissance in nursing. *Nursing.* 4 (25): 12-13.

Pfeil M (1994): Role of nurses in promoting complementary therapies. *British Journal of Nursing.* 3 (5): 217-9.

Quinn J (1984): The healing arts in modern health care. *The American Theosophist.* 72 (5): 198-203.

Rankin-Box D (1993): Innovation in practice: complementary therapies in nursing. *Complementary Therapies in Medicine.* 1 (1): 30-33.

Rankin-Box D (1995): Competence in the clinical setting: issues in nursing practice. *Complementary Therapies in Medicine.* 3: 25-27.

Reid T (1994): Women's health. *Nursing Times* special publication. London: Macmillan Magazines.

Royal College of Nursing, Australia (1997): Position Statement: *Complementary Therapies in Australian Nursing Practice.* Canberra, Australia: RCNA.

Spencer M (1998): Natural path's glow of health. *Australian.* 9 September, 1998.

Stein D (1990): *All Women are Healers: A Comprehensive Guide to Natural Healing.* California: The Crossing Press Freedom.

Stevenson C (1992): Holistic power. *Nursing times.* 88 (38): 68-70.

Teschendorff J, Chew D (1993): East meets West: nurses learning complementary healing therapies. *The Australian Nurses Journal.* 22 (9):16-19.

Thurtle V (1994): Viable alternative? *Nursing Standard.* 8 (2): 52-53.

Tiran MD (1992): Complementary therapies: use with care. *Professional Care of Mother and Child.* 2 (1): 4-7.

Trevelyan J (1993): Fringe benefits. *Nursing Times.* 89 (17): 30-33.

United Kingdom Central Council (1994): *Complementary Therapies:* Position statement. London: UKCC.

Watson J (1985): *Nursing: Human Science and Human Care.* Connecticut: Appleton-Century-Crofts.

Willis E (1994): *Illness and Social Relations: Issues in the Sociology of Health Care.* Sydney: Allen & Unwin.

Wright SG (1995): The competence to touch: helping and healing in nursing practice. *Complementary Therapies in Medicine.* 3: 49–52.

APPENDIX 4.1

Choosing a complementary therapies course: what should you consider?

Why choose a complementary therapy course?
Examine your personal reasons for wanting to do a course. Do you:
a) Want to use complementary therapies in conjunction with your nursing skills?
b) Want to develop a new career?
c) Want to develop your own self-awareness?

   If any of these is the case find out/do the following:
a) Do you need to be a registered nurse?
b) How long is the course?
c) How much is the course? Does it appear good value for money? Is payment required prior to commencement of the course?
d) How does the course compare with others?
e) Is funding available from your employer or another source?
f) Have you explored the implications/potential for implementing the complementary practice in your clinical environment? Have you discussed this with your manager?
g) Does the course accept anyone, regardless of aptitude or prior qualifications, with the money to pay the fees?
h) Does the course offer competent clinical supervision? Is case-study work a part of the course?
i) Visit the institution offering the course and speak to the lecturers prior to starting.
j) Request a detailed prospectus and ensure that the content is appropriate for your role as a nurse.

   Where possible discuss potential courses with colleagues who have qualified in this field. Avoid correspondence courses unless adequate clinical supervision is provided.

Course content and standing—consider the following:

1. Which professional associations will you be able to join when you have completed the course?
2. Which of those associations are accepted by health funds so that clients of their members can receive rebates for treatment?
3. Does any government legislation affect the therapy in question, e.g. regulation of premises where acupuncture is practised?
4. In summary, ensure that where appropriate the course includes:
   a) supervised practice
   b) anatomy, physiology, pathology and pharmacology
   c) a practical and theoretical examination
   d) a holistic approach
   e) supervised clinical practice
   f) counselling, communication and self-development skills training
   g) appropriately qualified lecturers
   h) support for the trainee therapist
   i) a sensible tutor/pupil ratio
   j) basic management and business skills
   k) postgraduate skills updates offered by school or association.

Prepared by Royal College of Nursing UK, Dept of Nursing Policy & Practice, Complementary Therapies in Nursing Forum and adapted by Pauline McCabe to suit the Australian context.

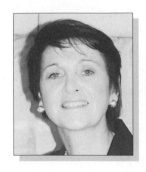

JUDITH LANCASTER
Bachelor of Arts/Bachelor of Laws (Hons), Master of
Bioethics, Diploma of General Nursing, Graduate Certificate
in Legal Practice, Graduate Certificate in Higher Education,
admitted as a solicitor to the Supreme Court of New South
Wales.

Lecturer, Faculty of Law, University of Technology, Sydney.

Judith is a nurse and a lawyer who graduated as a registered general nurse from St Vincents Hospital in Sydney. Her experience in the nursing profession spans 15 years in Australia and overseas. She undertook a combined Arts/Law degree as a mature age student, graduating with first class honours in 1991, and was admitted as a solicitor of the Supreme Court of New South Wales in 1992. Judith is currently employed as a lecturer in the Faculty of Law, University of Technology in Sydney, where she teaches health care law and business law. She recently completed a master's degree in bioethics. Her dissertation examined ways to increase the number of organ donations in organ transplant programs. Judith plans to commence doctoral work in 2000.

Legal and ethical aspects of complementary therapies and complementary care

INTRODUCTION

In recent years, changes in public attitudes towards the maintenance of personal health and wellbeing have generated unprecedented demand for access to a range of complementary therapies in both the preventative and the treatment contexts of health care. Along with this demand goes the expectation that health care professionals will be familiar with and incorporate appropriate complementary therapies into treatment regimes in order to provide a broader and improved range of health care strategies and patient care. In turn, there are now new legal and ethical considerations for nurses and other health care professionals who find themselves in unfamiliar territory when the inevitable question arises of how best to deal with a particular situation.

This chapter aims to identify the legal and ethical issues most likely to arise when complementary therapies are incorporated into nursing care, by examining the regulatory framework in which practitioners must operate.

THE REGULATION OF COMPLEMENTARY THERAPIES

The most significant aspect of the regulation of health care in Australia is the diverse range of regulatory controls operating. The federal constitutional model of government, with legislative powers divided between the Commonwealth and the States, increases the degree of regulatory complexity. In the case of 'conventional therapies' or those therapies administered within the rubric of scientific medicine, a plethora of regulatory machinery exists.

However, there are fewer regulations governing complementary therapies. Consequently, individual practitioners and other health care professionals engaged in performing and delivering complementary therapies, find themselves operating with far less professional certainty than that enjoyed by those operating strictly within the realm of conventional health care. As a result, the regulatory vacuum is slowly being addressed as the benefits of complementary care as a valuable health care strategy are increasingly acknowledged by mainstream health care authorities such as the Therapeutic Goods Administration, the Departments of Health in the various states, the nurses registration boards and the Royal College of Nursing, Australia. Regulatory controls fall into four broad groups: statutory law, common law, public complaints mechanisms and statutory and voluntary self-regulating associations.

1. STATUTORY REGULATION

The strict regulation of orthodox health care provides significant safeguards for patients and their carers. In contrast, the exclusion of many, if not most, complementary therapy modalities from formal regulation has denied those wishing to partake of such therapies and their carers a similar range of safeguards. While only a small number of specific complementary therapists, such as chiropractors and osteopaths, are formally regulated, others are regulated indirectly.

Thus, a number of complementary therapies are regulated through the operation of existing legislation governing individual aspects of health care such as that regulating the manufacture, storage and administration of drugs (*Therapeutic Goods Act* 1989 (Cth); *Narcotic Drugs Act* 1967 (Cth); *Poisons and Therapeutic Goods Act* 1966 (NSW) and individual state drug laws) or by virtue of the fact that they are administered by health care professionals already subject to statutory regulation such as nurses, doctors, pharmacists, physiotherapists and other allied health professionals.

The function of statutory regulation is to provide for the formulation of rules and regulations to which practitioners can refer as a guide to acceptable professional practices. It also serves as a formal framework for the setting of education, registration and disciplinary requirements. For example, in order to qualify for registration as a general nurse, mental retardation nurse or a psychiatric nurse in New

South Wales one must have completed a course of training and hold a recognised diploma, certificate or other award signifying successful completion of that course at a recognised institution in New South Wales in which a law providing for the registration of nurses is in force (section 19 *Nurses Act* (NSW), 1991). Under section 43 the Board is empowered to establish codes of professional conduct setting out the rules of conduct to be observed by accredited nurses in carrying out the practice of nursing. Formal complaints against registered nurses fall within the provisions of sections 44, and section 45 sets out procedures that must be followed by the Board in regard to complaints.

Similar regulatory provisions apply to chiropractors and osteopaths. In order to qualify for registration in New South Wales, chiropractors and osteopaths must be: above the age of 18 years, of good character, have completed a prescribed course of training and hold a diploma, certificate or other academic award or passed an examination arranged by the Board (sections 9, 10, and 11 *Chiropractors and Osteopaths Act* (NSW) (1991). Under section 27, the Board is empowered to establish codes of professional conduct containing rules of conduct to be observed by registered chiropractors and osteopaths. Formal complaints against registered chiropractors and osteopaths fall within the provisions of section 28, and section 32 sets out the conditions under which practitioners can be suspended from practising. Other jurisdictions have either the same or similar requirements.

2. COMMON LAW REGULATION

Common law is known in legal circles as 'judge-made law'. Unlike statute law, which comprises written sets of rules and regulations enacted by parliament, common law is developed in the courts on a case-by-case basis. This means a previous case can set a precedent for judgment in future, similar cases. Although common law liability can arise under both civil and criminal law, common law has most relevance for health professionals. In the health care context civil law actions can be brought in 'contract' or 'tort'.

A contract encompasses the rules that regulate business relationships such as the sale of goods, partnerships and insurance. Tort law, otherwise known as civil law, deals with wrongful activity that can arise in conjunction with or independent of a breach of contract, a crime or the violation of another person's equitable right. In other words, tort law deals with wrongful behaviour on the part of an individual that culminates in harm or is an intrusion to another.

CONTRACTUAL LIABILITY

The escalating costs associated with providing health care and the increasing tendency for individuals to want to take an active role in decisions concerning their health and wellbeing, have seen the concept of the patient as a consumer of health care services emerge. As a result, the civil actions in contract against health carers are now considered an appropriate way of seeking compensation for breaches causing loss or injury.

Contractual liability is most likely to arise in the health care context as a claim under consumer protection law. The most common category of claim is likely to be one concerning misleading or deceptive conduct in representations made to a patient by a health professional. Under section 52 of the *Trade Practices Act* 1974 (Cth) (TPA) it is an offence for a corporation to engage in conduct that is misleading or deceptive or is likely to mislead or deceive. Mirror legislation has been enacted across the individual states of Australia to recompense patients of hospitals, nurses, doctors, dentists, physiotherapists, chiropractors, osteopaths and other health care professionals whose non-corporate status places them outside of the provisions of the TPA (see Table 5.1.).

Table 5.1: Table of statutes

Chiropractors and Osteopaths Act (NSW) 1991

Consumer Affairs and Fair Trading Act (NT)1990

Fair Trading Act (NSW) 1987

Fair Trading Act (Qld) 1989

Fair Trading Act (Vic) 1985

Fair Trading Act (WA) 1987

Fair Trading Act (Tas) 1990

Health Care Complaints Act (NSW) 1993

Health Complaint Act (ACT) 1993

Health Rights Commission Act (Qld) 1991

Health Services (Conciliation and Review) Act (Vic) 1987

Health Services (Conciliation and Review) Act (WA) 1995

Narcotic Drugs Act (Cth) 1967

Poisons and Therapeutic Goods Act (NSW) 1966

Therapeutic Goods Act (Cth) 1989

Trade Practices Act (Cth) 1974

Misleading statements concerning the need for certain treatments or procedures, the adequacy and proficiency of the treatments or procedures and their risks and benefits can all fall within the definition of misleading conduct under consumer protection legislation. Similarly, failure to disclose pertinent information may constitute misleading or deceptive conduct ,or conduct likely to mislead or deceive.

Under consumer legislation a range of compensatory remedies is available to consumers who can establish that a breach of the consumer protection provisions has occurred. Any action taken under these provisions will not act as a bar to other claims of negligence under civil law providing the claimant is not seeking compensation twice for the same thing.

LIABILITY IN TORT

A tort is a civil wrong that arises from a relationship between two parties that is remedied by a compensatory award of damages. Tort actions against health care professionals commonly fall within one of two categories—battery and negligence.

Battery
Battery, commonly referred to under the more general heading of assault, is a trespass to a person who is touched against their will. An action in battery arises out of a violation of individual autonomy and is based on the principle of autonomous entitlement of all persons. Battery occurs where there is an intention to carry out a treatment or procedure on a person in circumstances where that person has not given consent or has otherwise withdrawn their consent. For example, a patient who requests that a particular treatment regime such as massage be discontinued can sue the therapist if the request is ignored. Battery can occur and compensation may be awarded by a court even if the person does not sustain any physical injury and is not aware of the unlawful interference at the time it occurred. It is sufficient that the unlawful act took place without consent.

Negligence
Negligence encompasses the notion of causing harm to another person by failing to take reasonable care. It can arise out of acts that result in harm to a person, or failure to act where harm results. This translates into doing what a reasonable nurse would not do in the same or similar circumstances, or not acting in a manner expected of a reasonable person. Three elements must be proved, on the balance of probabilities, for an action of negligence to succeed. These elements are a duty of care, a breach of that duty and physical and/or financial harm resulting from the breach.

DUTY OF CARE

A duty of care is based on the establishment of a close or proximate relationship between the parties. In the health care context a duty of care arises whenever a therapeutic relationship is established. A therapeutic relationship is one that exists between a health care practitioner and a person seeking advice or treatment in the course of that relationship. The therapeutic relationship is the same regardless of whether the practitioner is delivering conventional or complementary therapies or a combination of the two.

The defining principle of the duty of care is known as the *'neighbour principle'* and was set out in the landmark case of *Donoghue v Stevenson* (1932) AC 562, commonly referred to as the snail in the bottle case. The *'neighbour principle'* holds that one must take care to avoid acts or omissions that might foreseeably harm another person. 'Foreseeable harm' is any injury or damage that might reasonably be expected to result in the particular circumstances. For example, a nurse-complementary therapist administering herbal medication in conjunction with a conventional medication must take care to avoid potential interactions with the conventional medication. Care must also be taken to avoid using undiluted or strong concentrations of essential oils directly on the skin as this could cause a skin reaction or chemical burn.

STANDARD OF CARE

The standard of care is also derived from the *'neighbour principle'* which requires health care professionals to perform professional tasks to the same standard as that expected of an ordinary skilled professional with the same level of experience. The standard does not require that a practitioner display extraordinary skills and expertise but that they exercise the ordinary level of skill expected of a competent person professing to have the same skills.

The process of establishing the standard of care derives from the English case of *Bolam v Friern Hospital Management Committee* [1957] (1 WLR 582), which holds that acting in accordance with established professional standards acceptable to a responsible body of practitioners in that profession will satisfy the standard expected. This is known as the *'Bolam test'* and although it is still used to establish the standard of care in medical negligence cases in English courts, it no longer automatically applies in Australia. In 1992 the High Court of Australia, ruling in the case of *Rogers v Whitaker*

(1992) (175 CLR 479), changed the approach taken in the Australian jurisdiction. The *'Bolam test'* is no longer applied in cases concerning failure to warn of risks, and will not necessarily be applied in negligence cases arising from other medical contexts such as those concerning treatment and diagnosis.

While examining the issue of informed consent in *Rogers v Whitaker,* the High Court of Australia, criticised the *Bolam test* for its tendency to focus on what a reasonable body of professional opinion would expect from a reasonable practitioner in the circumstances, instead of considering what a reasonable patient should expect of a reasonable practitioner. The case of *Rogers v Whitaker* changed the perspective from which the standard of care is established away from a focus on professional opinion of how much information should be provided to a patient, in favour of a focus on a patient's right to be informed of the material risks.

A material risk is one that a reasonable person in the patient's position is likely to consider significant, or one that a practitioner should be aware that the particular patient would consider significant. In other words, the implication of *Rogers v Whitaker* is that health professionals are expected to be perceptive and communicate clear accurate information to those with whom a professional relationship has been established. The *Rogers v Whitaker* case makes it clear that health professionals are required to respond to the particular patient.

To safeguard themselves against the possibility of a patient claiming they have not been given adequate information, the nurse needs to be perceptive about the specific needs of each particular patient and the specific needs generated by that patient.

Although the principle from *Rogers v Whitaker* is confined to the particular issue in question in that case (which concerned a failure to warn of risks), it is important to remember that it may apply in other treatment and diagnostic contexts, that is to conventional and complementary therapies.

What this means for practitioners of complementary therapies and for nurses practising complementary care, is that they will be required to satisfy the same standard of care criteria as health professionals engaged in the delivery of conventional health care at the same level of experience. At a practical level it means ensuring that patients are provided with complete and accurate information, professional advice and all relevant details and alternatives likely to be regarded by them as important and significant.

3. PUBLIC COMPLAINTS MECHANISMS

Complaints commissions

There are several ways in which complaints about health care and its administration can be pursued and resolution sought other than resorting to formal court actions. In most states and territories of Australia commissions or units have been established by statute to deal with complaints pertaining to all aspects of both public and private health care. In South Australia the health complaints office is located within the South Australian Health Commission and deals with complaints about the public health care system. In the other states, the various bodies and legislation they are established under are shown in Table 5.2.

Table 5.2: List of state health complaint bodies and the legislation under which they were established

- ACT Health Complaints Unit
  (Health Complaint Act (ACT) 1993)

- NSW Health Care Complaints Commission
  (Health Care Complaints Commission Act (NSW) 1993)

- Queensland Health Rights Commission
  (Health Rights Commission Act (Qld) 1991)

- Tasmanian Health Complaints Commission
  (Health Complaints Act (TAS) 1995)

- Victorian Health Services Commission
  (Health Services (Conciliation and Review) Act (Vic) 1987

- Western Australian Office of Health Review
  (Health Services (Conciliation and Review) Act (WA) 1995

The legislation establishing these statutory bodies provides for the commissioner or director, as the case may be, to receive, assess and refer complaints for conciliation, investigation or disciplinary proceedings before the appropriate registration board.

The ombudsman

The ombudsman in each state has the power to investigate complaints made about decisions made by public officials in public institutions. Complaints arising out of the provision of private health services or health professionals operating in a private capacity are outside the jurisdiction of the ombudsman.

In contrast to the broad authority vested in the various State Health Complaints Offices and Commissions to provide appropriate remedies, the ombudsman's powers are limited to making recommendations and reporting the matter to the Parliament when the recommendations are not complied with. Because of their limited scope for obtaining enforcement of practical remedies, the ombudsman is not as frequently utilised for health care complaints as the other complaints mechanisms.

All health carers should remember that the best way to prevent obvious problems from escalating into major complaints is to promptly address early expressions of patient dissatisfaction by openly discussing the matter while the problem is in its early stages. Failure to resolve problems as they arise usually leads to the involvement of public complaint mechanisms.

4. SELF-REGULATING ASSOCIATIONS

While the law serves to formally define the legal limits within which professional practice operates, statutory and voluntary self-regulation plays a major role not only in translating the law into understandable guidelines but, more significantly, in establishing and maintaining the ethical dimensions of health care. Professional boards such as nurses registration boards and the Chiropractors and Osteopaths Registration Board are multifunctional bodies, authorised by statute to direct the operation of the relevant profession. Generally speaking, these functions are served by the relevant board's power to register those who can satisfy registration requirements, institute disciplinary proceedings where questions concerning professional standards arise and suspend or terminate registration where indicated. Professional codes of conduct serve as guidelines to the level of expertise and the standard of behaviour expected within the particular profession. It should be noted that the purpose of health professional registration boards is to protect the public, not the health professional.

Complementary care with its emphasis on holism and encouraging patients to assume an active role in their own health management, challenges mainstream conventional ideas of health care. As a result, the struggle for recognition of complementary therapies and complementary care as beneficial strategies in patient care is resisted by mainstream regulatory bodies.

However, change appears to be under way with positive responses from official bodies being noted both in Australia and overseas. In the United States, the Office of Alternative Medicine was established by the Senate in 1992 for the purpose of promoting unbiased study and research into non-conventional treatments (Brooke, 1998). In 1995 the Royal College of Nursing, Australia commissioned an enquiry into complementary therapies in Australian nursing practice.

The report concluded that there was 'a strong view coming from the profession that the incorporation of complementary therapies into nursing practice has the potential to enhance the role of the nurse as healer' (McCabe et al., 1995). The recent action on the part of the Federal Government in bringing the regulation of complementary medicines under the Therapeutic Goods Administration (TGA) is a welcome acknowledgment of the therapeutic benefits of complementary medicines and the need to provide a legal and ethical framework for safe practice.

In a recent US case an osteopathic physician was refused cover under his professional indemnity policy when he was sued by a patient whose finger had to be amputated after the osteopath removed a wart with tea tree oil injections. The insurer argued that the professional indemnity policy contained a clause excluding cover where any drug not approved by the Food and Drug Administration had been used. In declaring the clause legal, both the lower court and the Court of Appeal rejected the osteopath's argument that no approval was required because tea tree oil is not classified as a drug. The court ruling in this case established that the therapeutic purpose for which the substance was used was the deciding factor rather than the classification of the substance. (*Meza v Southern California Physicians Insurers Exchange,* (1997) Cal Ct APP 3rd District). For a list of cases refer to Table 5.3.

Table 5.3: Table of cases cited in the chapter

Bolam v Friern Hospital Management Committee (1957) 1 WLR 582
Donoghue v Stevenson (1932) AC 562
Meza v *Southern California Physicians Insurers Exchange,* (1997) Cal Ct APP 3rd District
Rogers v Whitaker (1992) 175 CLR 479

Notwithstanding these recent responses, the practice of complementary therapies and complementary care from a legal and ethical perspective remains in the developmental stages. Consequently, it is difficult to predict with any degree of certainty the extent of legal risk involved and the full range of ethical expectations. Nevertheless, liability risk is ever present and those health professionals looking to practise complementary care should observe a few essential guidelines including the following:

- Ensure that all patients are provided with accurate and complete information to enable them to make informed choices. Include clear details about all significant side-effects and complications that can arise from the therapy.

- Provide clear explanations of the nature of all procedures/treatment and how it will be given.

- Provide the person with up-to-date information about available options and alternatives. Always clarify with the person what the complementary care or therapy is expected to achieve and the function it will serve in the overall treatment regime. Make sure that the person never participates in a care regime with unrealistic expectations.

- Prepare patients for the possibility that their condition may not improve immediately and that, in fact, it may initially decline. It is important to ensure that patients are given full details of the planned treatment regime and the expected outcome.

- Evaluate the risks associated with the therapy to be administered and ensure that the patient is informed of them. Written consent is required for major procedures, that is procedures that have potentially significant consequences for the patient, but oral consent is usually sufficient otherwise. It is important to keep accurate, succinct records of all information supplied. It is wise to seek written consent in situations where there are significant risks of material harm or where there is reason to believe the consent being given may be the subject of dispute at a later stage.

- Always familiarise yourself with your employer's workplace policies. These should indicate whether the practice of complementary care falls within the scope of the employment contract. It is important that health professionals do not practise outside the scope of their employment, not only for the purpose of observing the conditions required by their employment contract but also to protect themselves from being excluded from indemnity under the employer's insurance cover as was the situation for the physician in the Meza case discussed earlier.

- Health professionals should be aware of the limit of their professional skills and experience and refer to colleagues and other health professionals as appropriate.

These guidelines apply equally to conventional care, however it is particularly important for complementary therapists to follow them because complementary therapies and complementary care may not be understood as well as treatment regimes associated with conventional care.

It is important for nurses who wish to practise as complementary therapists to ensure not only that their registration remains current but that they inform the Nurses Registration Board of their intention to so practise. In circumstances where registration has lapsed, to claim or imply registered status is an unauthorised use of qualifications for which the Board is authorised to impose specific penalties (section 40 *Nurses Act* (NSW) 1991). Section 40 also requires that the authority of the Board be sought for any use or claim of entitlement to use documents, title or status in or in relation to registration or enrolment as a nurse. While it is clear that registration under nurses acts carries authorisation for nursing practice involving conventional treatment and care, it is not so clear as to whether or not authorisation can be assumed to automatically extend to the practice of complementary therapies. That being so, it is essential to consult the relevant state Board before proceeding to practise complementary therapies either alone or in conjunction with conventional care.

CONCLUSION

Increased responsibilities now attach to nurses and other health professionals as the benefits of complementary therapies and complementary care and the possibilities they offer for improved health care strategies are acknowledged by a growing number of official bodies. However, fear of litigation or disciplinary action should not be a reason to restrict the practice of complementary care. It would be unfortunate if the rules and guidelines created to ensure safe practice and benefit patient care were to deny access to the contemporary health care strategies that are available. It would also be unfortunate if policies, guidelines and legislation were so prescriptive as to discourage nurses from exercising their judgment in the flexible and fluid manner that is so essential to sound patient care and is so much a part of the competencies that nurses exercise on a daily basis.

A better approach is to see the law and official policy documents as protective devices that guide safe practice and ensure the maintenance of high standards of patient care. Knowing what is required and practising in accordance with legal and ethical standards is the key to professional confidence and stability.

REFERENCES

Brooke PS (1998): Legal risks of alternative therapies. *Registered Nurse.* 61 5: 53–58.

McCabe P, Ramsay L, Taylor B (1995): *Complementary Therapies in Relation to Nursing Practice in Australia, Discussion Paper No.2.* Canberra: Royal College of Nursing, Australia.

Nurses Act (NSW) (1991).

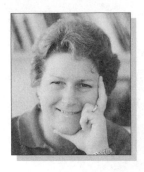

BEVERLEY TAYLOR
RN, RM, MEd, PhD, FRCNA, FCN (NSW)

Foundation Professor of Nursing, Southern Cross University

Beverley began nursing in 1968 in Tasmania and has been employed full time in the profession ever since, as a clinician, teacher and researcher. Her main interests are in all spheres of holistic nursing and she is the editor of the *Australian Journal of Holistic Nursing*.

Chapter 6

Research issues in complementary therapies and holistic care

INTRODUCTION

Complementary therapies in health care are therapeutic modalities or activities that complement and augment orthodox approaches. Holistic nursing and midwifery practice is a comprehensive way of being, knowing and doing in the delivery of nursing and midwifery care, which may include the use of complementary therapies. Although complementary therapies and holistic nursing and midwifery practice are often seen as being related, they are not the same and one does not necessarily guarantee the presence and effects of the other. Nurses and midwives may use a kitbag of strategies and therapies and still work in reductionistic, non-human-centred ways. In other words, they can choose to use complementary therapies in clinical and fragmented ways, devoid of interpersonal connection.

Complementary or natural therapies used in nursing and midwifery practice to augment patient care can be grouped into categories such as traditions of healing, therapeutic use of self, physical and energy therapies. Traditions of healing therapies include aromatherapy, acupuncture and reflexology. Therapeutic use of self includes humour, therapeutic and healing touch and visualisation therapy. Energy therapies include meditation, guided imagery and music therapy (RCNA Position Statement, 1997). All of these therapies make claims for patient wellbeing and healing, which can be tested and explored through research approaches. In health care settings, research is essential, because 'there is increasing pressure to evaluate the benefits and risks of all treatment and diagnostic modalities' (Meppem et al., 1997).

Since it became 'trendy', holism is interpreted in a number of ways. For example, for some people, holism involves thinking of humans as bio-psycho-social and spiritual beings and trying to care for them as complete beings (Benner, 1984; and Ferguson, 1976). Other people interpret holism as recognising and incorporating spiritual perspectives of care (Hetzel, 1991; Janiger and Goldberg, 1993; Keegan, 1994; and Thompson, 1994) and/or relating to people as open energy systems (Brennan, 1987; Brennan, 1993; and Rogers, 1970). For others holism is synonymous with the use of natural and complementary therapies, which augment personal health regimes and health care practices (Dossey et al., 1995). Lastly, when 'holism' is mentioned to some people, they associate it with a certain amount of 'new age rhetoric' and rituals, such as personal awareness strategies, 'alternative' living, ecological protection, rainbows, dolphins, and weekend market products, such as drums, dream catchers and crystal wind chimes. Any of these interpretations of holism can exist in various combinations and be of greater or lesser significance for the person espousing them. All of them are, and will remain, unsubstantiated if they are not subjected to research methods and processes. Holistic nurses may use a combination of these interpretations in their work and claim that they are practising holistically because they fulfil certain criteria of holism.

Over the last two decades there has been a growing interest in complementary therapies in Australian health care (Willis, 1984 in McCabe et al., 1995) and this has been reflected in Australian nursing and midwifery settings as patients demand complementary therapy options in their care management plans. Australian nursing and midwifery practice has responded to consumer demands with policies and courses guiding the use of complementary therapies. Policies have been produced by the Royal College of Nursing Australia, the Registration Boards of New South Wales, Western Australia and Victoria, the New South Wales Nurses Association, the Australian Nursing Federation, the Australian College of Holistic Nurses and the Holistic Nurses Association of New South Wales. Tertiary courses and units in complementary/natural therapies and naturopathy being accessed by nurses and midwives are established at Southern Cross University, Monash University, Victoria University of Technology, and LaTrobe University and several private providers now offer bachelor degrees in naturopathy.

Australian nurses' and midwives' interest in holistic nursing and midwifery began when American scholars Newman (1979), Rogers (1970) and Watson (1988) legitimised spiritual and human energy field perspectives of care through their writings, admitting to nursing and midwifery practice the possibilities of caring for humans as complete biopsychosocial and spiritual beings. The ideas caught on so strongly that holism became enshrined in tertiary nursing and midwifery curricula, rapidly becoming the catchcry of Australian nursing and midwifery clinicians, academics, managers and researchers (Taylor, 1995). *The Australian Journal of Holistic Nursing* is a refereed journal that publishes the research and practice experiences of holistic nurses and midwives, and includes papers on the use of complementary therapies. Although complementary therapies feature in the journal, it does not imply that they constitute completely the practice of holistic nursing.

In summary, nurses and midwives face the challenges of using complementary therapies 'holistically', that is, they need to be aware that holistic care is not necessarily guaranteed by simply using therapies as adjuncts to their usual activities. In addition, even with all the interest and advances in complementary therapies and holistic nursing and midwifery, there is still much to be done to improve the validity of both through research. The next section examines nursing and midwifery research in relation to the use of complementary therapies.

NURSING AND MIDWIFERY RESEARCH AND COMPLEMENTARY THERAPIES

Many nurses and midwives shy away at the mention of research, even though they do not need to be convinced that it is essential for their practice. Although I cannot hope to include all the issues, methods and processes of research in this chapter, I can address the potential for validating the use of complementary therapies through nursing and midwifery research. Where possible, references to assist nurses and midwives to set up their own projects are included.

RESEARCHING WHOLENESS AND COMPLEXITY

Holism is a difficult concept to understand and apply and critics have been eager to point out its shortcomings in general as well as in nursing, midwifery and health care. The arguments are:
- that holism is complex and almost impossible to conceptualise and apply (Adorno in Schanz, 1986; Bohm, 1980; Smith, 1988; and Williams, 1988)
- that it really only amounts to trendy new age rhetoric (Bruni, 1989; and Williams, 1988)
- that it is overly optimistic and idealistic and individualistic (Kramer, 1990; and Owen, 1995)
- that it has no sociopolitical conscience (Bruni, 1989; Kermode and Brown, 1995; Madjar, 1987; and Popper, 1974).

Holism is also rejected by critics who reject spiritual perspectives (Sobel, 1979) and the existence and effects of the human energy field and systems (Beyerstein, 1997). Opposition to holism is also based on opposition to the use of natural and complementary therapies with which it is deemed to be synonymous (Coward, 1993; and Green, 1997).

A close examination of the criticisms shows that it is relatively easy to find fault and shortcomings with understanding and applying holism because the concept is so immense and complex. The all-inclusive and intricate nature of holism combine to create an almost fathomless pit of ideas, options and applications, so there is little wonder that it can be criticised from all angles and perspectives. Paradoxically, the immensity and complexity of holism also make it ideal for research, because so many facets appear, all of which are open to scrutiny. Holistic health care is an especially rich field for research, because it involves inquiry into the human condition as it strives for wholeness and wellness. Within the broad band of holistic health care we find nursing and midwifery, and for the purposes of this chapter we will assume that the inclusion of complementary therapies in these disciplines denotes clinicians' intention to practise holistically.

How can the human mind capture complexity through research? The usual answer to this question has been a quantitative one, such as: 'If you take each small part of a puzzle and separate it from the whole of its context, you can capture complexity through rigorous observation and analysis'. A researcher making a response of this nature would most likely come from a school of thought known variously as the empirico-analytical, scientific or quantitative paradigm. A problem arises instantly from this response. For example, if holistic care values the immensity, complexity and wholeness of human existence, and it espouses non-reductionist ways of viewing people, how can complexity be captured without dividing humans into phenomena, issues, segments, units and sub-units of inquiry?

All aspects and entities within the known universe consist of wholes, and they combine into one continuous and vast realm known to human consciousness. Apart from claims of rare moments of cosmic awareness, there can be no way of knowing everything as a whole at any one time. Human inquiry must limit itself to exploring manageable parts of the puzzle of the greater whole, but it does not always have to resort to focusing in on the smallest parts, nor does it always have to separate those parts from their context. The decision about how small to reduce the piece of the puzzle and whether to allow it to remain context-bound, depends on the types of questions being asked and the methods for finding the answers. In other words, some research will of necessity reduce itself down to small parts such as energy, enzymes, nuclei and cellular organelles, while other research will view the puzzle from a wider lens and look at human phenomena, experiences, interactions and outcomes. There is no hierarchy of greater to lesser inquiry, there is only difference relating to the best way of researching according to the questions asked and the knowledge sought.

My answer to the question of how to capture complexity generally and in holistic health care in particular, can be described as: use whatever inquiry approaches, methods and processes are necessary to give the answers to the puzzle of the greater whole and the smaller wholes contained within it. If the question requires a close, even subatomic focus, that is fine. If the question requires a broad, universal focus, or any place in between the very small and the very large, that is also fine. However, in capturing the complexity of holistic nursing, midwifery and health, research should always attempt to maintain the integrity of the whole, keeping parts of inquiry within the context of the whole of the human condition. In other words, if I am researching the effectiveness of a complementary therapy it will always be in relation to all aspects of the humans experiencing it, that is, in the context of their biopsychosocial and spiritual wellbeing. Do not separate the therapy from the humans experiencing it and fail to reconnect them.

EVIDENCE-BASED PRACTICE

Evidence-based practice was the dictate of the 1990s, and it is as it seems—practice based on research. The evidence-based practice movement grew out of the need for practice to have clinical validity and not to be the perpetuation of treatments which had little or no research credibility. Shorten and Wallace (1997:22) defined evidence-based practice as 'the conduct of health care according to the principle that all interventions should be based on the best available scientific evidence'. Research into complementary therapies fits well within an evidence-based practice framework given the need to prove they are effective and safe. This does not mean anything new for nurses and midwives who recognise the value of research.

The evidence-based practice movement is merely a banner for a systematic approach for ensuring that research stays in practitioners' minds as an essential part of their practice. Nurses and midwives seeking to use complementary therapies in their practice need to be aware of the various implications for their use, including why and how they are used, how they work, and their demonstrated effects. Not only will this information assist nurses and midwives to learn more about specific therapies, it will also point to where research is needed.

TYPES OF NURSING AND MIDWIFERY RESEARCH

There are many types of nursing and midwifery research that differ according to their intentions, methods and processes. The problem for beginner researchers is that the types of research vary so greatly and it is difficult to know where to begin and how to proceed. Let's begin with some background information of what research is, what it intends, the means it uses, and the outcomes it achieves, to enable you to get a grasp on the whole of this activity we call nursing and midwifery research.

The intention of research is to 're-search', or examine issues by asking questions, usually in an area of interest. Research attempts to find new knowledge and confirm previously held knowledge and assumptions which it can show to be 'true'. The researcher's intentions are reflected in the research question and expressed as the aim and objectives, such as: 'This research aims to examine the effectiveness of lavender aromatherapy on insomnia for people with dementia', or 'This research aims to explore, with carers, their perceptions of the effectiveness on insomnia of lavender aromatherapy for their relatives with dementia'. Specific objectives then follow which outline the detailed intentions of the overall aim.

Many methods are used to gather information, for example, double blind trials, surveys, interviews and participant observation. The methods chosen often reflect the type of knowledge required. For example, a double blind trial may be used when scientific knowledge of an absolute type is required from which effects can be predicted and other cases can be generalised. Using the previous example, this might mean that two types of aromatherapy treatments are randomly assigned to two groups of people with dementia, in such a way that neither the carers nor the researcher are aware of the specific research intentions or the purported therapeutic effects of a particular treatment. Conversely, unstructured interviews may be used when scientific knowledge of a relative type is required from which insights can be gained when findings resonate with readers. For instance, carers of relatives with dementia could be encouraged to discuss their subjective experiences in relation to the effectiveness of a certain type of lavender essential oil used to aid their relative's sleeping patterns.

Both methods are scientific in the sense of *scientia*, meaning knowledge, because they are applied and analysed systematically and carefully to produce new or amended knowledge. In the case of the examples used here, however, the former method would have greater influence with readers who require some objective proof of the effectiveness of the aromatherapy. Research methods must be stringent so that the knowledge they produce is reliable and truthful and completely devoid of lies, deception and conjecture. Therefore, research processes use criteria for ensuring rigour or trustworthiness so that veracity or truthfulness can be established. A thorough account of these processes can be found in the relevant sections in Roberts and Taylor (1998:81–84 and 172–175) and Bowling (1997:130–138).

Research processes are *how* methods are applied and how people in the research relate to one another in order to achieve the research intentions. Processes include consideration of the use of language, the degree of involvement and collaboration of people and the 'ownership' of the project. For example, quantitative researchers tend to refer to people in the research as 'subjects', whose involvement should be limited carefully to avoid bias, and who have no rights of ownership of the research. Qualitative researchers refer to people in the research as 'participants', who have varying degrees of involvement and collaboration, and who thus have some ownership of the research. The differences in these research processes reflect the intentions and methods of two main approaches—quantitative and qualitative research. Although there are some shortcomings in dividing all research into two main types, the quantitative and qualitative distinctions help readers to grasp the main overarching concepts of research.

The first section of this chapter introduced the main parts of a research project. To learn more about how to construct a research proposal further reading is needed (see, for example, Roberts and Taylor (1998:213–248) and seek the help of someone who has research experience. In the next section I will describe the differences between the two research types to help you understand why certain choices must be made when doing research for specific purposes.

QUANTITATIVE AND QUALITATIVE RESEARCH

The simplest way to think about the difference between quantitative and qualitative research is to imagine that the former is concerned with numbers and mathematics and the latter is concerned with words and language. Qualitative approaches to research grew out of a need to explore human questions and issues in different ways from those offered previously

In summary, quantitative research seeks absolute and certain knowledge, in which people are removed from their contexts for the purposes of objective scrutiny. Quantitative research uses deductive inquiry to start with broad inferences and observations stated as hypotheses, to move towards specific instances. The results of quantitative research claim predictive ability and generalisability by being statistically significant. Strict measures of rigour are applied to ensure that projects are valid (actually measure what they intend) and reliable (can be retested for comparison), so that results can be trusted as 'truthful'. As a general rule, the reverse is true of qualitative research, which values relative knowledge, of a context-dependent, inductive, non-predictive and non-generalisable type, whose results are verified as trustworthy according to the degree to which they resonate with participants and provide insights for them.

RESEARCH METHODS

'Methods' refers to the means by which information is collected and analysed. Data collection in quantitative research is managed by the use of surveys, questionnaires, controlled trials, structured observations and interviews (Roberts and Taylor 1998:145–166). Information can be collected in qualitative research by many methods including archival searches, artistic expression, case studies, fieldwork, group processes, interviews, journal keeping, literature searches, member checks, observation, participant observation, photography, storytelling and videotaping (Roberts and Taylor, 1998:175–184). Each of these methods has specific structures and processes that must be adhered to carefully to ensure their success. Potential researchers need to be aware of what they are in order to use them effectively. Data analysis methods vary according to the type of research, but in general, quantitative data are analysed by mathematical means and qualitative information is analysed by language-based means. Knowledge and practice in research analysis ensures that results are valid and this only comes with tenacity and experience.

Quantitative and qualitative research approaches can be used to explore complementary therapies in nursing and midwifery practice, either separately or in combination. The decision about which approach to use depends on the questions asked and the methods and processes required. Questions about precise relationships between variables, using objective methods and processes to reduce human bias require a quantitative approach. Questions focusing on areas of human interest, in which subjectivity is welcome and essential, can be answered using a qualitative approach. A combined approach can be taken if the researcher wants to do 'a bit of both'.

EXAMPLES OF TYPES OF STUDIES AND THEIR FINDINGS

The amount of research into complementary therapies is substantial and growing within the fields of nursing and midwifery as well as generally. There is an urgent need for a national database to contain the magnitude of the research, especially in the face of criticisms that little or no research exists. Although this paper cannot list all, or even many, of the projects, it is important to know that many studies have been done and are of great use to readers. For example, there have been studies in healing touch (Hover-Kramer, 1996), therapeutic touch (Krieger, 1976; Kramer, 1990; and Smyth, 1995) and aromatherapy (Mills, 1997; MacMahon and Kermode, 1998, and Clarke, 1999). These projects and others use a variety of quantitative and qualitative approaches to explore specific areas of interest.

Hover-Kramer (1996) documented quantitative studies into healing touch in relation to enzyme changes, relaxation effects, immune system changes, pain relief, childbirth preparation and wound healing. Kramer (1990) compared therapeutic touch and casual touch in stress reduction of hospitalised children. Krieger (1976) demonstrated the bioenergetic changes in the hands of therapeutic touch healers and in vivo human haemoglobin. Clarke (1999) used aromatherapy to reduce stress in a haemodialysis unit, MacMahon and Kermode (1998) examined the effects of aromatherapy in a dementia unit, and Mills (1997) described the positive outcomes of implementing aromatherapy in a busy and stressful clinical environment. Why not locate and read some of these articles to familiarise yourself with how and why to do research?

MANAGEABLE RESEARCH IN CLINICAL PRACTICE

In clinical research it is important only to 'bite off what you can chew'. Projects should be modest at first, centring on one problem or set of problems in a focused, systematic manner. Always begin with a clarification process in which you become very clear about what you want to research, why, and how. These deliberations will allow you to express your research questions or area of interest, aims and objectives, and methods and processes. All of these aspects come together in a succinct research plan which contains certain sequential steps according to the type of research method you are using. Manageability is important in any research. Researchers need to bear in mind many issues including the size, design, cost and duration of the project to ensure they can cope with the intentions of the research, choose the most appropriate methods, and keep to budget and on time.

EVALUATION OF CURRENT PRACTICES

If you are currently using complementary therapies in your practice, it makes a lot of sense to focus in on your own work to begin research projects. For example, you could use your own documentation and record keeping to create case studies and to set up larger projects involving various degrees of experimentation and description. Patient feedback about the usefulness of therapies is very important. If you are not keeping detailed records of your work you could begin soon, with research validation in mind.

A good starting point is to remember that practice and research can happen at the same time. This is especially so if you reflect systematically on your practice with the intention of improving it constantly. Although you may feel confident in your clinical skills, you may need to spend some time reading about research approaches and putting small manageable projects into operation as soon as you can. You will discover that research is like any other new venture—it gets easier with more practice.

Compile a list of good books and the names of researchers you can call on as often as you need to ensure that you make a start in researching your practice. Introduce yourself to academics in the institutions named in this chapter, and ask if they will help you set up projects. The chances are that they are looking for clinical connections and will be happy to collaborate with you. Read about research into complementary therapies in journals and books, and study how they are set up and what results come out of them. These steps may build your confidence in knowing you are capable of managing research projects and disseminating the results of your own work.

CONCLUSION

This chapter introduced complementary therapies in holistic nursing and midwifery practice and the possibilities of doing research into complementary therapies. Quantitative and qualitative research were described as research approaches and methods and applications were made to complementary therapies. The chapter concluded with suggestions for manageable research in clinical practice, beginning with the evaluation of current practices. I wish you well in your practice and in validating complementary therapies through research.

REFERENCES

Benner P (1984): *From novice to expert: Excellence and power in clinical nursing practice.*
Menlo Park: Addison-Wesley.

Beyerstein B (1997): Why bogus therapies seem to work. *Skeptical Inquirer.* September/October
21(5): 29-34.
Bohm D (1980): *Wholeness and the Implicate Order.* London: Routledge and Kegan Paul.

Bowling A (1997): *Research Methods in Health: Investigating Health and Health Services.*
Buckingham: Open University Press.

Brennan BA (1987): *Light Emerging: The Journey of Personal Healing.* New York: Bantam Books.

Brennan BA (1993): *Hands of Light: A Guide to Healing Through the Human Energy Field.*
Toronto: Bantam Books.

Bruni N (1989): Holism: A radical nursing perspective. Paper presented to National Nursing Theory
Conference South Australian College of Advanced Education. In: Koch T (ed.) *Theory and practice;
An evolving relationship.* Sturt: The School of Nursing Studies.

Clarke D (1999): Advancing my health care practice in aromatherapy. *Australian Journal of
Holistic Nursing.* 6(1): 32-38.

Coward R (1993): The Myth of Alternative Health. In: Beattie A, Gott M, Jones L and Sidell M (1993):
(eds) *Health and Wellbeing: A Reader.* Houndmills: Macmillan.

Dossey B, Keegan L, Guzzetta C and Kolkmeier L (1995): *Holistic Nursing: A Handbook for
Practice.* (2nd ed). Gaithersburg: Aspen.

Ferguson MC (1976): Nursing at the crossroads: Which way to turn? A look at the model of nurse
practitioner. *Journal of Advanced Nursing.* 1(3): 237-242.

Green S (1997): Pseudoscience in alternative medicine. *Skeptical Inquirer* September/October
21(5): 1-5.

Hetzel R (1991): *The New Physician: Tapping the Potential for True Health.* Victoria: Houghton
Mifflin Australia.

Hover-Kramer D (1996): (ed.) *Healing Touch: A Resource for Health Care Professionals.* Albany:
Delmar Publishers.

Janiger O and Goldberg P (1993): *A Different Kind of Healing: Doctors Speak Candidly About
Their Successes with Alternative Medicine.* New York: Putnam Books.

Keegan L (1994): *The Nurse as Healer.* Albany: Delmar Publishers.

Kermode S and Brown C (1995): Where have all the flowers gone?: Nursing's escape from the radical critique. *Contemporary Nurse* 4(1): 8-15.

Kramer MK (1990): Holistic Nursing: Implications for Knowledge Development and Utilisation. In: Chaska N (ed.) *The Nursing Profession: Turning Points.* St Louis: CV Mosby, pp. 245-254.

Krieger D (1976): Healing by the laying on of hands as a facilitator of bioenergetic change: the response of in vivo human haemoglobin. *Psychoenergetic Systems* 1:121-129.

MacMahon S and Kermode S (1998): A clinical trial of the effect of aromatherapy on motivational behaviour in a dementia care setting using a single subject design. *Australian Journal of Holistic Nursing* 5(2):47-49.

McCabe P, Ramsay L, Taylor B (eds) (1995): *Complementary Therapies in Relation to Nursing Practice in Australia.* Discussion Paper No. 2. Deakin, ACT: Royal College of Nursing, Australia.

Madjar I (1987): Wholistic nursing: Challenges, options, choices. Paper presented at the Challenges Options Choices International Conference. New Zealand Nurses Association: Rotorua, pp. 1-12.

Meppem M, Crawshaw K, Wilson A, Adrian A (1997): The health department position: complementary therapies in mainstream medicine. *Lamp* 54(6):8-9.

Mills J (1997): Aromatherapy on the ward: The whiff of 'de-stress'. *Australian Journal of Holistic Nursing* 4(1):41-44.

Newman MA (1979): *Theory Development in Nursing.* Philadelphia: FA Davis.

Owen M J (1995): Challenges to caring: nurses interpretation of holism. *Australian Journal of Holistic Nursing* 2(2):4-14.

Popper KD (1974): *The Open Society and Its Enemies: Volume 2: Hegel and Marx.* London: Routledge and Kegan Paul.

Royal College of Nursing, Australia (RCNA) Position Statement, (1997): Complementary Therapies in Australian Nursing Practice. Deakin ACT: Royal College of Nursing, Australia.

Roberts K and Taylor B (1998): *Nursing Research Processes: An Australian Perspective.* Melbourne: Nelson ITP.

Rogers ME (1970): *The Theoretical Basis of Nursing.* Philadelphia: FA Davis Company.

Schanz HJ (1986): Naivety and cynicism: The total of the totalitarian. *Acta Sociologica.* 29(2):149-157.

Shorten A and Wallace M (1997): Evidence based practice: The future is clear. *Australian Nursing Journal* 4(6):22–24.

Smith MJ (1988): Perspectives on wholeness: The lens makes a difference. *Nursing Science Quarterly* 1(3):94–95.

Smyth D (1995): Healing through nursing: the lived experience of therapeutic touch. *Australian Journal of Holistic Nursing* 2(2):15–25.

Sobel DS (1979): *Ways of Health: Holistic Approaches to Ancient and Contemporary Medicine.* New York: Harcourt Brace Jovanovich.

Taylor B (1995): Of holism and other conundrums. (editorial) *Australian Journal of Holistic Nursing* 2(2):3.

Thompson P (1994): *Finding Your Own Spiritual Path: An Everyday Guidebook.* Minnesota: Hazelton.

Watson J (1988): *Nursing: Human Science and Human Care. A Theory of Nursing.* New York: National League for Nursing.

Williams K (1988): World view and the facilitation of wholeness. *Holistic Nursing Practice* 2(3):1–8.

Willis E (1984): The Role of Alternative Health in Australia In: McCabe P, Ramsay L, Taylor B (1995) (eds) *Complementary Therapies in Relation to Nursing Practice in Australia.* Discussion Paper 2. Deakin, ACT: Royal College of Nursing, Australia.

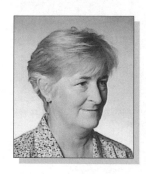

SUE CECHNER
RN

Aged care coordinator for the United Protestants Association, North Coast Region, New South Wales

Sue's varied nursing career has included being charge sister of a plastic surgery unit, sister-in-charge of the cardio-thoracic unit and a nurse educator at the Royal Melbourne Hospital, and working in several London hospitals. She spent ten years on Bougainville Island in Papua New Guinea. For the past eighteen years Sue has been involved in the aged care industry, previously as a director of nursing (in Victoria and NSW). She combines her role in aged care with facilitating workshops and running a successful complementary therapies practice. Her career path has been very important to Sue and she feels fortunate to have been able to combine several of her interests—educating health care workers, aged care (in particular, dementia care) complementary therapies, communication with the family unit, taking control of health and wellbeing, stress management and research into the use of complementary therapies in nursing.

Careers and opportunities: complementary therapies and future nursing

INTRODUCTION

In the current climate of commercialisation and the seduction of science, it is clear that the medical field is far from immune to the pressures of commerce and economics. As a result, the character of health care, and the role of various health care workers is ultimately changing and adapting, either within the current health field, or in alternative areas.

The past decade has seen a strong contingent of nurses choosing to progress and diversify for a number of reasons, including an attempt to attain job satisfaction following disenchantment with the current health system. In addition, it has also become necessary to diversify in order to meet the increasing needs of a general public that is searching for holistic health rather than treatment of symptoms. Some nurses have felt the need to unite personal philosophies and lifestyle with health care. The changes in society mean the potential for nurses, and nursing, in complementary therapies is increasingly positive, immense and certainly diverse.

FROM HUMBLE BEGINNINGS

My personal career journey took me from registered nurse and charge sister in a cardio-thoracic unit, to nurse educator, director of nursing in a number of aged care facilities, aged-care coordinator of hostels, and finally to nurse practitioner–complementary therapist in a holistic practice. It was some ten years ago that I realised the deficiencies in modern medicine, after I returned to my original training hospital and the open heart ward where I had been charge sister. During a period of hospitalisation I was made aware of the changes that had occurred in nursing from a patient's perspective. The technical care was excellent but the emotional support was non-existent. In ten days I was not touched, nor did anyone actually listen to me. Not until I returned home to my family did I feel the care and attention that I needed in order to recover. It is with observations and experiences such as these, that many nurses are searching for alternatives. James Gordon MD (1996) also experienced a similar situation and comments that:

> *The many voices of personal experience have an authority which is compelling all of us to question all received medical truths and to search for and demand new techniques and new models of care.*

James Gordon's statement led me to recall the time when I was a director of nursing in a nursing home on the North Coast of NSW in 1990, making my morning rounds. I was frequently told by the residents about the wonderful foot massage or lavender bath they had received; rarely was I told about the shower or the great enema. I often thought, at that time, that it would be wonderful for nurses to integrate technical, physical and emotional support for those in their care.

I saw the advantages of using aromatherapy in aged care after I attended a workshop run by Sunspirit. My physiotherapy aide bought lots of lovely little bottles of essential oils from the Sunspirit trade display. Then came the problem—what to do now? How do we use them? We went to the local hairdresser who provided us with an endless supply of perm solution bottles and we made massage blends. We thought we were achieving great results, and the residents enjoyed their massages. It was only later we learned that essential oils should be kept in coloured glass containers. From these humble beginnings we embarked on, what I believe, is one of the greatest movements in nursing.

I decided we needed to know more about essential oils. Eventually we found an aromatherapist who came to Ballina to run a series of training sessions. A range of staff members from Ballina nursing homes and hostels, registered nurses (RNs), assistants-in-nursing (AINs) and diversional therapists attended these sessions. Several of us carried on to attain aromatherapy and/or reflexology diplomas. Other nurses in the region were impressed by what we were achieving.

In the Northern Rivers region where I live and work, we are now integrating technical, physical and emotional support for those in our care, despite a little opposition. It is still common to encounter nurses and staff who feel that complementary therapies are 'nonsense' and who are resistant to change. Importantly though, most doctors are supportive, administration is positive and works with us, and relatives appreciate the personalised attention their loved ones receive. One nursing home in the Region is beginning to address the needs of relatives, particularly those of dying residents.

To combat any opposition, it has been vital to network and support each other through groups such as the Aromatherapy Network Group and the Holistic Nurses Interest Group. An example of our support network is the use of video conferences to link nurses in Lismore and Grafton, enabling them to discuss success, problems, and related issues. Several complementary therapy modalities are now used in a range of health care settings in the Region—in private practice, midwifery, community care, aged care and specialist units in acute care.

A HOLISTIC MULTIDISCIPLINARY PRACTICE

The medical practice in which I work is a holistic one. Thus, private practice is an avenue that is open to many nurses wishing to diversify into complementary therapies. I have been a member of the team since 1993, originally as the only complementary therapist working with five doctors. Recently the practice became truly holistic. Visitors are often pleasantly surprised to see my name and the therapies I practise listed alongside the doctors' qualifications. We now have five therapists working from the practice. These therapists have various backgrounds and previous professions. Two are nurses.

The objective of the health centre is **wellness,** the philosophy being that each member of the health team works with clients to achieve education, wellbeing and growth. In this practice the nurse practitioner is an equal and valuable member of a dynamic team and is perceived to be credible, reliable and confident. The integration of orthodox medicine and complementary therapies, in my experience, has been most successful. Patients/clients like to know, that as well as being a complementary therapist, I also have a traditional nursing background. This gives them confidence. In addition to using reflexology on their feet I also take their blood pressure or give an injection. The collaborative practice model acknowledges that no one modality can effectively cover all areas of health, therefore, it was important to form a network of colleagues who can work together in a supportive environment.

One of the primary objectives of this particular health centre, and indeed others, is to reduce health costs. In our practice we predict that results from the growing number of holistic practices will reduce rates of heart attack, stress, hospital visits and medication usage. If this is the case, the government could then allocate valuable health dollars to areas that require urgent attention. To the consumer, at first glance, the cost of complementary therapies appears significant. However, when considering the possible consequences of disrupted work, taking medication, stress and loss of income, it becomes an appealing alternative. Complementary therapy nurses must take opportunities to raise awareness of the positive benefits of their therapies. Nurses frequently underestimate the true value of their work and may not charge appropriately for their services. Asking people to pay for services is difficult for nurses coming from a salaried background. A business management course is invaluable to assist them to develop financial skills.

There are other examples of private practices on the North Coast of NSW. Gaye, a registered nurse for 32 years, who has lived and worked in a farming community for 20 years, recently established a complementary healing centre in her community in response to a number of factors. Her personal success with complementary therapies and her experience in working with a homeopath led to a desire to respond to a genuine need in the community. Feelings of discontent with the present health system (for example, serving patients meals which she knew were not nutritionally sound) and the belief that orthodox medicine provides short-term cures without dealing with the cause of the disease or problem, also motivated Gaye. She asserts that the move towards complementary therapies as an option for the community began when general practitioners in the area changed their charging methods from bulk billing under Medicare to fee-for-service. The public wanted value for their dollar and started to take responsibility for their own wellness and this seems to be an international phenomenon.

Subsequently, the range of clients utilising Gaye's centre represents a cross section of the farming community, from older farming families and pensioners, to young families and members adopting alternative lifestyles. However, Gaye's success was not without its problems and she has been confronted by some stalwarts in the medical community who feel they 'possess' their patients and that their decisions are unquestionable.

Sue Enzer, a registered nurse and reflexologist, is another successful complementary therapy nurse who specialises in midwifery and maternity reflexology. In addition to working as a practitioner in Sydney, she also lectures and runs workshops in Australia and overseas. Her course is endorsed by the Australian College of Midwives. Dye (1992:100) claims that:

> *There are many midwives using complementary therapies with great success, and as more and more positive results are being recorded, more and more [nurses] are attending courses to learn, increase their knowledge or develop their skills further.*

INDUSTRIAL NURSING

Commercialisation has increased awareness of complementary therapies as companies promote natural wellbeing. Companies such as the Body Shop and Drake International support stress management and relaxation. Therefore, there are opportunities for industrial nurses to incorporate complementary therapies into their traditional roles. Although not particularly prevalent on the North Coast of NSW, industrial nurses are employed by businesses and corporations to reduce stress, workers compensation claims, employee dissatisfaction and work related problems. In the past, industrial nurses were employed to cater for first aid needs, but their roles have expanded as employers place greater emphasis on preventing injury and illness and promoting 'wellness' programs. Industrial nursing is an exciting area in which a complementary therapy nurse could be very successful.

HOSPITAL PRACTICE: LONG TERM AND ACUTE

Registered nurses working in acute hospital settings are also experiencing changes in terms of care and support of patients. Despite the pattern of nurses moving to other fields of employment, there are possibilities for nurses to integrate complementary therapies into acute care settings. Ramsay, in a personal communication in 1999, suggested that complementary therapies are best suited to long-term units, such a palliative care, midwifery (including antenatal) and aged care. It is in these environments that nurses can develop a relationship with clients and integrate complementary therapies into individual management plans. It is often more difficult to implement these therapies in acute care settings because of the lack of acknowledgment of the benefits of complementary therapies within the orthodox medical field. Having said that, the growing recognition of the benefits of complementary therapies will certainly increase their level of use in the acute area in the future.

In acute hospital environments the traditional model of nursing is the most common at this stage. Nurses seeking to introduce complementary therapies into acute care settings are being confronted with difficulties in obtaining approval from hospital management and in implementing policies and procedures. However, the Nurses Registration Boards of New South Wales, Victoria and Western Australia have developed guidelines for the use of complementary therapies in nursing practice. These policies recognise the valuable interventions and therapeutic approaches of the various complementary modalities and formalise standards for their use. The Nurses Board of Victoria defined complementary therapies or interventions as, ' . . . treatments that are aimed at a more holistic approach to healing' (NBV, 1996, revised 1999).

It is promising for the future careers of nurse-complementary therapists that nurse registration boards are aware of the growing interest in, and use of complementary therapies. This indicates that career options for nurses using complementary therapies in hospitals are indeed available and will become increasingly viable. It is imperative that nurses interested in this particular option read the Australian Nursing Federation (ANF) Policy Statement on *Complementary and Alternative Therapies* (ANF, 1996) and the ANCI *Code of Professional Conduct for Nurses in Australia* (Australian Nursing Council Inc., 1995).

Therapeutic interventions, whether complementary or orthodox, should be supported by written policies and protocols which are endorsed by the employing facility (Nurses Registration Board of NSW, 1998). At present, however, many hospitals allow essential oils to be supplied and used by patients during their hospitalisation, which presents risks because quality assurance, documentation of the oils used and evaluation of the effects of the oils are lacking. As these risks are identified it is possible to assume that hospitals will be placed in the position of altering their practices and allowing registered nurses to extend their fundamental qualifications to include an integration of traditional and complementary therapies.

In some current situations, and indeed in the future, it will be common for the nurse to utilise complementary therapies in acute care. Their potential to reduce stress and anxiety in the hospital situation is fantastic. I often advise clients on the use of complementary therapies pre-operatively, during hospitalisation and post-operatively. In particular, aromatherapy could be invaluable in acute care. Essential oils may be used for a range of purposes from simply providing a pleasant aroma in a hospital, through acting as a calmative, to providing specific relief from various conditions. According to Worwood (1995:302):

> *Nurses are quite right to think that essential oils could certainly do away with many of the problems they see in hospitals every day, but aromatherapy is more than application of essential oils, and to use essential oils correctly and safely, nurses may have to revise their thinking on how healing actually works.*

It is imperative that nurses receive appropriate training. In the near future we may begin to see standardised training for nurses.

Although complementary therapies are not being used in hospitals in a consistent manner nationwide, some areas are implementing appropriate and exciting programs. Possibilities for the complementary therapy nurse within the acute hospital setting need not be limited to the role of consultant employed by individual clients.

In summary, although some hospitals are incorporating complementary therapies into their care plans, the use of these therapies has not been formalised on a general level. At this stage there have not been many opportunities for nurses to specialise in complementary therapies within a particular hospital. However, it is with anticipation that we look toward the future, and implementing complementary therapies on a broad base. For the nurse considering career options, it is feasible to assume that the role of complementary therapies will improve and, without a doubt, increase, in the acute hospital. Hence, it remains essential that nurses document their skills and practices in complementary therapies.

The Australian government responded to recommendations from the Therapeutic Goods Administration Review (TGA) (1996) by establishing a new Complementary Medicines Advisory Committee. The TGA will also pursue the accreditation of complementary medicinal practitioners with state and territory governments (Australian Food News, 1996). Senator Christopher Ellison (1996) also stated that '57% of the Australian population currently use complementary medicines ..', which means that the government needs to address the role of complementary therapies in health care, including standards of training and services. These moves by the government can only benefit the nurse-complementary therapists and raise their profiles.

HOSPITAL IN THE HOME

As a direct result of the commercialisation of health care and hospitals, the early discharge of patients has paved the way for exciting career options for nurses who wish to incorporate complementary therapies into their roles. For example, individuals recovering from illness or operations have many needs following hospitalisation that have often been overlooked in the past. It is possible to establish a business which either identifies and caters for these needs specifically, or works collaboratively with general practitioners.

Recently my daughter underwent major surgery which necessitated an overnight stay in hospital. We utilised aromatherapy pre-operatively to prevent infection; during hospitalisation to reduce stress, anxiety and pain; and post-operatively in the home. This recovery period was very successfully dealt with using complementary therapies. We were able to use various therapies to assist with scarring, pain, swelling and general wellbeing. It is my belief that services such as these would be received extremely positively by people who are often overwhelmed by their experiences and who are looking for something to meet their needs.

Furthermore, there are numerous possibilities for using complementary therapies in 'hospital in the home' situations, an option that would work very successfully for complementary therapy nurses. Not only would they be working with particular therapies to heal the body, mind and spirit, but they could use their traditional training to aid their work and assist client recovery. For those individuals who wish to manage their illness, injury, or disease at home, the 'home hospital' offers them the opportunity to incorporate a range of healing modalities into their care.

AGED CARE

On the North Coast of NSW, the aged care facilities are far more open to complementary therapies than are the acute hospitals. There are more career opportunities for the complementary therapy nurse in aged care because of the recognition of the value of such therapies. In a number of nursing homes and aged care facilities, policies have been established to ensure the safe use of complementary therapies. Therapies are included in the care plans of individual residents, and complementary therapies are used as a funding tool. This progressive approach has motivated many nurses to undertake training in a range of complementary therapies such as aromatherapy and reflexology. Registered nurses are expanding their training and increasing their employment opportunities by participating in complementary care as the value of touch and 'one-on-one' care is acknowledged.

I have been involved in establishing and facilitating the Northern Rivers Aromatherapy and Complementary Therapies Research Network. The objectives of this network are to document the effectiveness of complementary therapies to ensure their ongoing and increased utilisation. Projects such as this will improve career opportunities for nurses.

COMMUNITY-BASED PROJECTS

Community-based projects are also presenting opportunities for nurses to expand into complementary therapies in many interesting and diverse ways. The Community and Aged Care Packages in Ballina, NSW, established a specific program for clients. A nurse, with aromatherapy and reflexology training, was employed expressly to introduce complementary therapies into the program. The project is enjoying success; both clients and management have noted the benefits.

The Far North Coast Carer Respite Centre, another community based project, offers opportunities in complementary therapies by providing regular 'carer indulgence days'. On these days carers are invited to choose from a range of complementary therapies to reduce their stress and allow them to continue their difficult caring tasks. A similar project, the Holiday Respite Program, was developed for carers and their dependents. Both these programs cater for the needs of the participants and provide opportunities for particular complementary therapy nurses to share their knowledge and skills. Complementary therapy nurses are invaluable in these projects because of their understanding of the pressures and issues involved in caring for sick relatives. Their traditional background and nursing education allow them to empathise with and advise carers and provide information about the disease and associated problems.

Government initiatives such as the 'Staying on Your Feet' program is another area where the nurse-complementary therapist is able to take an increasing role in the health care arena. Working as a nurse-complementary therapist, I participated in this program and have subsequently been able to educate and increase public awareness of the benefits of integrating traditional and complementary therapies. Nurses moving into the complementary therapy field are responsible for promoting their skills and therapies and should be involved in small community projects in order to increase their role in the community.

PUBLIC SPEAKING

As a complementary therapist and registered nurse I am frequently asked to attend functions as a keynote speaker. I address women's groups, service groups and conferences, and provide inservice training. It is interesting to note that I have been asked to speak as a complementary therapist more often than I was as a nurse. Part of the role of the complementary therapy nurse is to encourage individuals to be responsible for their own wellness and growth. Through guest speaking I am able to promote this concept as well as the benefits of complementary therapies. Having nursing qualifications helps because audiences respond positively to the credibility of a traditional health care background.

Although I often present papers at seminars and conferences on a fee for service basis, I also volunteer my time to talk to small groups such as foster parents and head injuries groups and I gain the most from these particular public speaking occasions. As a complementary therapy nurse I am committed to helping and healing others; if I can provide that assistance to those who give themselves so tirelessly and constantly to others, I feel I am achieving my goals.

HEALTH PROMOTION AND PREVENTATIVE CARE

The promotion of wellness and responsibility for self-health also includes roles in sports injury prevention, and working with youth to address current health and welfare issues. Opportunities for the complementary therapy nurse arise in these areas as we look toward the future and the trend towards prevention becoming the 'norm'.

In general, the complementary therapy nurse should advocate illness prevention and health promotion, which includes personal lifestyles and may involve utilisation of the 'home hospital'. Being received as sincere and genuine is important for nurses and complementary therapists. In order to enjoy these attributes they use complementary therapies with their family, pets and friends. One of the greatest benefits to me has been my personal wellness and the fact that my children have integrated complementary therapies into their lifestyles. The advantages recognised for nursing are also present for the nurses and their families—increasing positive communication and creating a happier, more harmonious lifestyle.

GETTING STARTED

The best way to begin is by using a range of complementary therapies for family and personal use. I have used many modalities from the outset with my family. My eighty-three year old mother uses massage blends to alleviate arthritic pain, my daughter used various essential oils to assist her through school and university, and my son, a jackaroo, used oils as first aid and for his chronic fatigue syndrome.

There are a number of points to consider when getting started:
- Try several therapies yourself to find one/s you feel comfortable using.
- Read as much information as you can.
- Attend trade displays and expos.
- Attend a short course to establish and consolidate your interest.
- Follow this with more intensive training.
- Network with other complementary therapy nurses.
- Study and practise.

CONCLUSION

In conclusion, complementary therapies have made my working life fun. As a director of nursing I was respected in the community. I am still respected, but also have a diverse range of friends, acquaintances and colleagues from a variety of backgrounds, age groups and areas. The world of nursing has expanded my horizons and taken me a long way from the young nurse who left the Royal Melbourne Hospital. Careers and opportunities for nurses in complementary therapies are diverse and far reaching. As we look toward the future and set goals for our careers we must not be limited by the institutions which dominate our training. There are myriad opportunities for nurses in this great, exciting area. I wish you well on your journey of discovery.

REFERENCES

Australian Food News (1996): Government Response to Recommendations arising from the Therapeutic Goods Administration Review. *www.ausfoodnews.com.au/flapa/pharmresponse.htm:* accessed July 1999.

Australian Nursing Council INC.(1995): *Code of Professional Conduct for Nurses in Australia.* Canberra: Australian Nursing Council INC.

Dye J (1992): *Aromatherapy for Women and Children.* Great Britain: CW Daniel Company Ltd.

Ellison, Senator Christopher (1996): *Australian Government releases major statement on drug regulation.* http://acupuncture.com/News/AustHerb.htm:accessed July1999.

Gordon, James, MD (1996): *Changing how we define medicine.* www.healthy.net/ library/articles/mindbodyconnectio/mbdefmed.htm: accessed July 1999.

Holistic Nurses Association of NSW (1998): *Policy on Complementary Therapies in Nursing Practice.*

Nurses Registration Board NSW (1998): *Complementary Therapies in Nursing Practice.*

Nurses Board of Victoria (1996, revised 1999): *Guidelines for Use of Complementary Therapies in Nursing Practice.* Melbourne: Nurses Board of Victoria.

Nurses Board of Western Australia (1996) *Guideline Statements for Use of Complementary Therapies in Nursing.* Perth: Nurses Board of Western Australia.

Worwood V (1997): *The Fragrant Mind.* Great Britain: Bantam Books.

Personal communications
Ramsay Lyn (1999): Lecturer Southern Cross University, New South Wales.

Section Two

Complementary therapies: some therapeutic approaches

OVERVIEW

Seven therapies or therapeutic approaches have been selected for in-depth discussion in this book. The therapies included have been selected because they are considered to be the most relevant to current Australian nursing practice. They are by no means the only complementary therapies being used by nurses and midwives but space precludes the inclusion of every therapy. Nutrition, aromatherapy, massage, relaxation therapies, therapeutic touch and healing touch, music therapy and animal-assisted therapy (pet therapy) are included. Nutrition heads the list because of its pre-eminent role in the onset of many diseases, and in their management and prevention. The information has personal as well as professional relevance for nurses and midwives, who need to consider diet as part of their own stress management and health promotion strategies. The remaining therapies are fairly well known. Aromatherapy, massage, relaxation therapies, therapeutic touch and healing touch, and music therapy are increasingly used by nurses and midwives. Up-to-date information is provided on these therapies. The role of animals in the healing process is perhaps less well known. Australians are great animal lovers and pet owners, and this therapy has been included because of increasing interest in, but a lack of information about, ways to incorporate animals into practice. Animal-assisted therapy is often taken for granted, yet research is increasingly validating the healing effects of caring for animals.

Section Two approaches complementary therapies not merely as therapies, but in a wider context as ways to improve quality of life, promote health, contribute to rehabilitation, prevent disease, and ease the critical transitions of those in the care of nurses and midwives. Complementary therapies provide ideal ways to achieve many of these aims that are basic to our role.

SELECTED COMPLEMENTARY THERAPIES

Chapter 8, **Nutrition as a complementary therapy,** sets the tone for complementary therapies as agents of healing and health promotion. Greg May, nurse-naturopath, combines careers in both these disciplines, and has a special interest in nutrition. He sets out the relationship between diet, health and disease with a particular focus on the aetiology of disease. The free radical theory and its relationship to a deficient diet is clearly explained. Certain groups in society, for example the elderly and pregnant women, are prone to nutritional deficiencies and suggested nutrition regimes are provided. Nurses are in a primary position to provide advice on healthy eating to their patients. This chapter provides basic nutrition information and a guide to sources of further information and education.

Chapter 9, **Aromatherapy,** was written by Margaret Meyer, registered nurse and qualified aromatherapist. Margaret discusses various aspects of aromatherapy, including its history, its application in nursing and midwifery, recent research into its use and educational approaches towards using it. Aromatherapy appears to be the complementary therapy of most interest to nurses and midwives. This chapter provides a thorough introduction to the subject. Some interesting case histories are included to demonstrate the practical benefits of aromatherapy in various situations.

Chapter 10, **Massage,** by Laurie Grealish and Angela Lomasney, covers another popular therapy that is often utilised in nursing and midwifery. As touch is fundamental to nursing, massage can be a valuable adjunct to almost any area of clinical practice. This chapter describes the basic techniques of massage and discusses the indications for massage. A comprehensive account of relevant research in the area is included. Case histories are a feature of this chapter.

Chapter 11, has been titled **Relaxation—the learned response** by its author to remind readers that, unlike the stress response, relaxation does not happen automatically. Judy Lovas is a consultant in the areas of complementary therapies and psychoneuroimmunology (PNI). She discusses the link between the mind and the body, and PNI research that now provides theoretical support for the use of various complementary therapies. Judy clarifies the findings about PNI and the relationship between stress, relaxation, the mind, and the feeling state. Simple exercises in relaxation, guided imagery and meditation are included to enable the reader to experience these states.

Chapter 12, **Therapeutic Touch and Healing Touch—nursing modalities for the new millennium** explores two related therapies. Jane Hall is the Director of Healing Dimensions, a nurse consultancy in health and education. The origin and development of Therapeutic Touch (TT) and Healing Touch (HT) by nurses makes an interesting introduction to what are contemporary nursing applications of ancient healing techniques. A considerable amount of nursing research is now available on these therapies, and examples are presented along with their application in nursing. Education programs are now available in Australia for the practice and teaching of TT and HT. These therapies are increasingly finding a place in the practice of nurses and midwives.

Chapter 13, **An introduction to music therapy,** was written by Tonia Plack, a consultant in the area of music in health care. Tonia uses music as a healing modality with individual clients and advises industry on the role of music in creating a healing environment. Music is another ancient therapy that is experiencing a renaissance as a contemporary healing modality. Music as sound waves and as evocation has many interesting effects on the body and mind. These effects can be negative as well as therapeutic. Music therapy is clearly explained and relevant research from various disciplines is used to support the discussion. Practical advice on different approaches to music therapy, from one-on-one to ambient sound, is offered.

Chapter 14, **Nursing and the role of animals,** introduces a complementary therapy which is not as yet well represented in the nursing literature. Kirsten James, a nurse-consultant on the integration of complementary therapies into the workplace, has been reading in this area for some years and presents a comprehensive review of the relevant literature. Animals can assist healing and wellbeing in numerous ways and they don't necessarily have to be 'pets'. Humans have related to animals for millennia, and in recent years researchers have begun to investigate what this relationship may mean in terms of human health. As well as summarising the literature about pet therapy, Kirsten provides guidelines for its application in nursing practice.

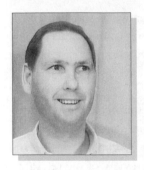

GREGORY MAY
RN, Accredited Naturopath, Bachelor of Naturopathy,
Graduate Diploma in Iridology, Certificate in Homoeopathy,
Graduate Diploma in Nutritional Medicine.

Current study: Graduate Diploma of Business Management

Greg has practised as a registered nurse and naturopath in both Victoria and Western Australia and possesses a wealth of knowledge and experience in the health industry. His particular interest lies in the ageing and degenerative process and he has also been strongly involved in community education. Greg was a regular guest speaker on Melbourne community radio station 3MDR and he continues to focus his attention on community education and awareness.

Chapter 8

Nutrition as a complementary therapy

INTRODUCTION

Nutrition is often overlooked in health care and viewed to as a non-scientific modality. The aim of this chapter is to demonstrate that nutrition does have a scientific base and is worthy of implementation in the prevention and treatment of disease, even in today's technological age. The chapter will provide health practitioners with a basic understanding of nutrition and the role it plays in health and disease. Nurses are often the first port of call in relation to health advice. The information in this chapter will assist them to enlighten those with whom they come into contact.

HISTORY

Documented nutritional deficiency diseases involving humans can be traced back to 1500 BC when journals written by Egyptians recommended the consumption of animal livers as a cure for night blindness (Ballentine, 1978). The active ingredient may not have been identified as vitamin A, but liver was effective nevertheless. It was not until 1912 that vitamins were identified, marking the first major step towards the recognition of nutrition as a science. Discoveries such as the structure of deoxyribonucleic acid (DNA) by Watson and Crick and the role of vitamins by Nobel Prize winner Dr Linus Pauling have paved the way for today's nutritional scientists (Wright, 1999).

Nutrition is an evolving science. New discoveries continue to be made and used to improve health, for example phyto-oestrogens, a group of plant chemicals with a similar structure to human sex hormones. Phyto-oestrogens possess demonstrated anti-cancer properties especially against breast and prostate cancer. Exciting new findings continue to emerge, and as this information becomes more readily available, nutrition will command a higher therapeutic profile.

NUTRITIONAL INFLUENCES ON THE AETIOLOGY OF DISEASE

Elements that affect cellular ageing

The basis of health is determined by the state of the cells, including the DNA. DNA is an inherited blueprint that instructs cellular activities. This genetic information is passed on from one generation to the next and remains constant unless mutations occur as a result of copying errors or breaks in molecule DNA. Nutrients have a profound effect at a cellular level in several ways. Nutrients provide nourishment, assist in energy production and affect the integrity of the DNA. Free radical damage causes mutations and cellular death. Free radicals are very reactive chemical products that are created as fuel is burnt in the presence of oxygen.

Anti-oxidants and nutrients protect cells from free radicals that are naturally produced by the body's metabolic processes. Excessive consumption of fried foods and exposure to toxins within our environment can increase the number of free radicals and compromise an individual's health status. Anti-oxidants are elements that have the unique property to donate an electron to the free radical, thereby inactivating it. Anti-oxidants come in the form of vitamins, minerals, enzymes and herbs, and can be found in the foods we eat and drink, especially fresh fruit and vegetables.

An inadequate level of anti-oxidants together with a high influx of free radicals may accelerate the degeneration and ageing processes. Such an imbalance can lead to:
- altered gene expression
- tissue and cellular damage
- immune dysfunction
- hormonal disorders
- neurological disorders.

Today's degenerative diseases

The free radical theory is not new, it has been well documented over the last few decades. The free radical theory proposes that most degenerative diseases, including heart disease, cancer, cerebral vascular accidents and neuro-degenerative diseases, as well as the ageing process itself, are a result of cellular damage due to free radicals. Indeed, at a cellular level, nothing is of greater importance than nutrition in order to achieve optimum health and longevity. Circulatory disorders, brain dysfunction and fatigue all have their beginnings with a poor nutritional status, and as a result, their treatment may include the modality of nutrition.

Circulatory problems

Nutrition plays an enormous role in the prevention and treatment of vascular disease. It has been well documented that a nutrient deficiency can result in structural changes and degeneration of blood vessels (Ames et al.,1993:7915) which not only affect the condition of the circulatory system, but the entire body. Such structural changes to blood vessels can manifest in a multitude of symptoms and ailments such as myocardial insufficiency, peripheral vascular disease, hypertension, cerebral insufficiency and varicose veins.

A study conducted in 1991 and reported in the *Clinical Science Journal,* demonstrated the effects of three anti-oxidant agents—vitamin C, thiopronine and glutathione—in hypertensive subjects. Not only did the study suggest that free radicals contributed to the development of hypertension, but also conveyed that anti-oxidants may well have a role in its treatment and management (Ceriello et al., 1991:739–742).

BRAIN AGEING AND NEUROLOGICAL FUNCTION

The brain is most susceptible to free radical damage due to several factors:
- The brain is an extremely active organ in which glucose is used at a very high rate that in itself results in high levels of free radical production.
- Brain DNA is very susceptible to damage due to its proximity to the generation of free radicals produced through energy production. It has been reported that brain mitochondria DNA has ten times more oxidative damage than DNA in the liver.
- Mitochondria DNA has fewer repair mechanisms, making it more vulnerable to damage than nuclear DNA.

The high levels of oxygen in and around the brain, and the fact that the brain creates an environment that is highly destructive to itself, produces an accelerated degenerative process leading to brain ageing and dysfunction. The need to supplement with anti-oxidants is therefore very clear. One extremely important anti-oxidant in relation to brain ageing is Coenzyme Q10 (Q10). Q10 is also an important co-factor that is essential to protect neural cells from oxidation and to maintain adequate energy reserves. Studies suggest that anti-oxidant action and preservation of mitochondrial function apparently provided by Q10 may protect from the free radical effect (Matthews et al., 1998).

The presence of high levels of free radicals in the brain environment, together with a low level of Q10 and other important anti-oxidants such as vitamin E, sets the stage for the development of neurological disorders. According to many well recognised medical research teams and leading research journals around the world, free radicals and abnormalities of oxidative metabolism play a significant role in the development of such neurological diseases as Alzheimer's and Parkinson's Disease, cerebral vascular disease and dementia (Tariot, 1994).

FATIGUE AND LACK OF VITALITY

Fatigue and decreased wellbeing are symptoms that are all too often expressed on a regular basis. Nutrition is an important element that should not be ignored in the treatment of stress and fatigue. In fact, nutrition has a significant impact on how we feel, and how we respond to our world.

Many foods consumed today lack the vitamins and minerals necessary for optimum health and vitality, because of over farming and erosion of soil. It was shown as far back as 1936 in US Senate Document 264, that soils and their crops were depleted of minerals, which resulted in mineral deficiency diseases (Wallach, 1997). This, together with modern day processing, storage and preparation of foods, can lead to loss of micro-nutrients (Buist, 1995b). It is possible to have a sub-clinical deficiency of essential nutrients with no obvious signs of disease other than a sense of reduced quality of life which may present in nonspecific ways such as a lack of vitality or even irritability.

Over the years there has been much debate about the Recommended Daily Intake (RDI) of vitamins and minerals. The two schools of thought in relation to RDI stem from the argument about when nutritional deficiency diseases become apparent. RDI is based on the smallest quantity of vitamins required to prevent nutritional deficiency diseases. It applies to a population as a whole and not an individual, and is based on the average health of the average person on an average day. The second school of thought is that health is not just the absence of disease but rather having optimal health and wellbeing. In order to achieve this greater level of functioning, a higher quantity of nutrients is required and therefore dosages exceed those of the RDIs.

It has been suggested that the RDI data is outdated and requires revision because sub-clinical deficiencies do affect the health and longevity of an individual and therefore must be addressed (Bland,1998).

Studies have demonstrated that marginal deficiencies of essential nutrients, including folic acid, pantothenic acid, vitamin C, iron, magnesium, potassium and zinc, may cause fatigue. Repletion of these nutrients will restore normal energy levels (Werbach,1993: 283).

INDICATIONS AND CONTRAINDICATIONS OF NUTRITIONAL SUPPLEMENTS

It has been stated time and time again that 'you can obtain all the nutrients you need by eating the four main food groups and it is not necessary to supplement'. This statement has confused the general population and even health professionals for a long time. The 1993 report of a study conducted by the Commonwealth Scientific and Industrial Research Organisation (CSIRO) Division of Human Nutrition, concluded:'anti-oxidants have a significant positive effect on heart disease. However, the level of vitamin intake necessary to achieve this protection would not be possible by diet alone.'This study lends weight to the importance of responsible nutritional supplementation (Buist, 1995b).

Anti-oxidants and other nutrients work as co-factors with their unique individual properties, in an attempt to maintain a biochemical equilibrium. Taking mega-doses of one vitamin thinking that it will rectify all one's health problems is certainly a mistake, and may even lead to ill health. The belief that if it is natural, it is not harmful, and in fact must be good for you, is a disturbing view and one that should be dispelled. Nutrients and medications may interact and deleteriously affect the health status of the individual. Table 8.1 describes the contraindications, possible drug interactions, indications for use and the recommended pharmacological dose (PD) of particular nutritional supplements. The pharmacological dose has a saturation level within the body that produces a therapeutic or pharmacological outcome, and as a consequence the dosage range is higher than the recommended daily intake (RDI).

Table 8.1: Indications for use, dose, recommended daily intake, contraindications and potential drug interactions of vitamins and minerals

Supplements	Indications	Dosage	Contraindications and drug interactions
Vitamin A	Essential for vision, healthy tissue, bone development, wound healing	RDI 5000 iu PD 10 000–100 000 iu	Avoid high dosages during pregnancy Neomycin reduces the absorption of vitamin A
B1 Thiamine	Fatigue, numbness in legs, calf tenderness, ataxia	RDI 1.5 mgs PD 100–500 mgs	Oral contraceptives containing oestrogen
B2 Riboflavin	Photophobia, eye burning and itchiness	RDI 1.8 mgs PD 10–500 mgs	Chloramphenicol interferes with B2
B3 Niacin	Muscle weakness, anorexia, skin eruptions, confusion, disorientation, neuritis	RDI 20 mgs PD 100–3000 mgs	Tetracycline increases niacin excretion
B6 Pyridoxine	CNS abnormalities, malaise, depression	RDI 3 mcgs PD 10–2000 mcgs	Cycloserine reduces B6 levels
Folic acid	Blood disorders, megablastic anaemia, GI disturbances	RDI 400 mcgs PD 400–10 000 mcgs	Anti-convulsants Methotrexate
B12 Cobalamin	Neuropsychiatric abnormalities, depression, Stiffness and generalised weakness of the legs	RDI 3.0 mcgs PD 10–2000 mcgs	Colchicine decreases the absorption of B12
Vitamin C (Ascorbic acid)	Loose teeth, wound healing, swollen and inflamed gums, prevents wound breakdown	RDI 45 mgs PD 100–10 000 mgs	Aspirin decreases serum levels of ascorbic acid

Vitamin E Tocopherol	Poor circulation, intermittent claudication, peripheral neuropathy	RDI 15 iu PD 15–1000 iu	Vitamin E may exacerbate hypertension when it is supplied in an oily form
Vitamin D	Poor bone structure, rickets in children, osteomalacia in adults	RDI 400 iu PD 400–100 000 iu	Interacts with the use of long-term anti-convulsants
Zinc	Maintains taste, smell and sight; necessary for hair growth; general immunity	RDI 15 mgs	Diuretics increase urinary excretion of zinc

Key

RDI	recommended daily intake
PD	pharmacological dose
iu	international units

NURSING AND NUTRITION: A POWERFUL THERAPEUTIC RELATIONSHIP

Clearly a distinct relationship exists between an individual's health and nutritional status. The nurse as a 'primary health care practitioner who is available as a first contact for a health problem' (McCabe et al., 1995) is therefore in an excellent position to provide information. In support of the nurse's role, various organisations such as the Australian Nursing Federation, Royal College of Nursing, Australia (RCNA), and the Nurses Boards in NSW and WA have developed policy statements about the use of complementary therapies, including nutrition, in nursing practice.

Studies have been conducted in order to provide guidelines for nurses to carry out a nutritional assessment and implement appropriate action. One nutritional assessment guide (Reilly, 1996) suggests nurses should:

- measure patient's weight and height and establish if weight is appropriate for height
- enquire about any recent weight loss and look for signs of fat and muscle wasting
- assess skeletal muscle strength (ask patient to squeeze your hands)
- assess respiratory function—look for effort of coughing and shortness of breath
- observe mobility
- observe wound healing and pressure sores

- observe for general mood, alertness and ability to concentrate
- ask patient about food intake
- check recent and current food intake
- ask about changes in appetite and avoidance of particular foods
- document current food intake using food charts.

The 1993 British Royal College of Nursing (RCN) paper entitled *Nutrition Standards and the Older Adult* is another such study. It was clear from this study that:

> *Many people were looking to the nursing profession to take a lead in screening elderly patients in hospital who were at risk of, or were already suffering from gross nutritional deficiency.*

(Watson, 1994:206).

Nutrition is also of great importance to individual nurses, as the nature of their profession can lead to nutritional neglect and susceptibility to ill health. It has been documented that shift work can affect metabolism and reduce motivation for maintaining good dietary habits, because regular eating patterns are difficult to establish. 'Shift workers also experience more frequent headaches, fatigue, stress, muscle pain, respiratory infection and general malaise' (Harvard Medical School, 1999). The relationship between nursing and nutrition is reinforced by the nursing profession itself, as is evident in the next section which cites nursing literature that emphasises the need for nursing involvement.

REASONS WHY NURSES SHOULD GET INVOLVED

- 'Nutrition plays a vital role in the recovery, health and life expectancy of transplant recipients' (Hasse, 1997).
- 'Poor wound healing and decubitus ulcers can signal the presence of protein, vitamin C and zinc deficiencies' (Morrison, 1997).
- 'The consequences of poor nutrition for elderly people are well documented in terms of susceptibility to infection, increased risk of developing pressure sores and a multitude of deficiency disorders which significantly reduce quality of life' (Watson, 1994:205).
- 'Nursing involvement in the identification and management of nutritional depletion is vital in the care of elderly persons' (Tierney, 1996:230).
- 'Poor nutritional status is associated with prolonged recovery from illness or surgery and increased health costs' (Lennard-Jones, 1992).

- 'Malnutrition is now recognised to be a frequent complication of hospitalisation' (Lennard-Jones, 1992).
- 'Improving nutritional status is associated with better clinical outcomes' (Tierney, 1996).
- 'Nurses should regard nutrition as making a positive contribution to treatment. Its success or failure is to some extent dependant on nurses' interest, knowledge, motivation, skill and understanding' (Holmes, 1993:30).
- 'Nutrition must be seen as a priority in a patient's treatment, as the success of all other treatments depend upon the individuals nutritional status' (Wallace, 1993:92).
- 'Optimal physical and cognitive function is greatly enhanced by good nutritional status' (Rosenberg and Miller, 1992).

COMMON NUTRITIONALLY DEFICIENT GROUPS: SUGGESTED TREATMENT APPROACHES

Institutionalised elderly

The nutritional component in the aetiology of any ailment or disease is often overlooked in the day to day management of the institutionalised elderly. A leading gerontological journal as recently as 1993, reported that 'elderly long stay hospital patients were grossly undernourished and their dietary intake did not satisfy basal metabolic demands' (Lipski et al., 1993). This is not a slur on the health system but rather an attempt to convey a new dimension to practitioners.

Nurses have a complex multifaceted role, one of those roles is that of client advocate (Kneisel, 1986:15). Nurses are in a position to ensure that the appropriate nutritional requirements of their clients are provided, and to educate regarding good nutrition and specific needs. The client will often adhere to the advice of the nurse as a close rapport usually exists between them, and it is because of this that nurses have a strong insight into their clients' health issues.

A commonality of health issues amongst the institutionalised elderly exists including:
- poor skin integrity and wound healing
- fatigue and lethargy
- altered mental state, which may present as depression, disorientation, aggression or poor cognitive function
- susceptibility to infection.

These ailments are often considered to be part of the ageing process and the true aetiology ignored. A low nutrient intake or drug interactions that affect the uptake or excretion of nutrients may result in changed health status. 'Malnutrition in hospitalised patients has been estimated to be as high as 20%–60%, and has been associated with increased morbidity' (Mion et al., 1994).

A regime to support treatment and prevention of the common health problems of the elderly should include supplements such as:
- Pantothenic acid, thiamine, vitamins A, C, E and zinc, which all have a strong influence on wound healing, as well as the ability to maintain skin integrity in the first place;
- B group vitamins (especially B12), vitamin C, magnesium, evening primrose, Coenzyme Q10, chromium and folic acid, which all combat fatigue, depression and poor cognitive functioning.

Pregnant women and pre-conception care

Nutrition plays an important role in the health of the mother and baby. The DNA integrity can be determined nutritionally prior to conception, therefore, good nutrition should be implemented for at least three months prior to conception. When the ovum and sperm unite, the genetic blueprint is laid down and these instructions of cellular reproduction may not be reversible. If one or both partners are nutritionally deficient, defective or inappropriate instructions of cellular division may result. The subsequent cascade of events may well lead to a life of ill health for the child.

An example of this particular situation can be seen with the nutrient folic acid. Folic acid is one very important nutrient that has been well documented in the prevention of neural tube defect, such as spina bifida (Buist, 1997c:1–2). A significant consequence of folic acid deficiency is an altered DNA metabolism, which affects the cells that proliferate most rapidly and has an enormous effect in times of rapid growth and development.

Vitamins and minerals are necessary for a vibrant pregnancy and a healthy child. A deficiency of certain vitamins and minerals may contribute to conditions such as hypertension, pre-eclampsia, low birth weight and, possibly, the risk of pre-term delivery. Not only is it advisable to supplement during pregnancy, but it is equally important to avoid certain foods and beverages, including alcohol and caffeine. Mothers consuming caffeine during pregnancy have a higher incidence of delivering a child with a low birth weight. Alcohol can affect the developing baby. Even mild alcohol ingestion during pregnancy is said to result in hyperactivity, short attention span and emotional lability in children (Gold et al., 1984:3).

In recent times herbal remedies have received a great deal of exposure in the media, including the herb ginger as an anti-nausea remedy during pregnancy (Buist, 1995a (3):53). Ginger may or may not be appropriate for every individual as it also contains other properties such as anti-clotting factors. Professional nutritional advice during pregnancy should always be obtained. Nutrients that can be used safely during pregnancy include thiamine, riboflavin, calcium, zinc, chromium, magnesium and essential fatty acids. The influences of these nutrients during pregnancy are as follows:

- Thiamine, riboflavin and chromium have a positive correlation with infant birth weight and size.
- Calcium is a mineral that should be doubled during pregnancy. Low dietary intake of calcium may be associated with pre-eclampsia and pre term delivery.
- Magnesium intake early in pregnancy may be directly associated with infant birth weight and size and is beneficial in the treatment of pre-eclampsia.
- Low maternal zinc has been associated with spontaneous abortion, premature delivery, and labour abnormalities.
- Fatty acids are beneficial for pregnancy induced hypertension. (Werbach, 1993:524-537).

Behaviourally challenged

In some circumstances nutrition can have a significant effect in the treatment of those individuals who are behaviourally challenged. The B group vitamins such as niacin, riboflavin and thiamine have a significant effect on mental wellbeing. A niacin deficiency can manifest as weakness, tremors, anxiety and depression. In severe cases the classical signs of acute psychosis may be apparent. Folate also has a role to play, together with B12. These two nutrients are intimately connected and a deficiency can result in neurologic and psychiatric sequaelae (Teodoro, 1998).

A field of nutrition that assesses mental disturbances in relation to the nutritional status of an individual is gaining recognition as a separate identity. Conditions such as depression, irritability and mood swings may be alleviated with the use of nutritional psychiatry. In using nutritional psychiatry, it is necessary to complete a nutritional assessment of the individual who presents with any behavioural or psychiatric difficulty. 'Nursing service has an important role in seeing that the client and family can provide additional information about food habits or problems that may affect client co-operation' (Davis and Sherer, 1994).

Once it has been established that there is a nutritional influence on psychological behaviour, an appropriate dietary regime can be implemented. Common vitamin deficiencies that may result in behaviour disorders and depression, are vitamins B1,

B6, B12 and C, as well as low levels of serotonin. The nurse should then work 'in close co-operation with the clinical nutritionist or dietitian and physician to co-ordinate medical and nutritional management of the patient's illness into overall nursing care' (Lewis, 1986).

COST OF NUTRITIONAL SUPPLEMENTS TO THE INDIVIDUAL AND SOCIETY

People often speak of supplementation of minerals and vitamins as an expense rather than an investment in their health. A sense of wellbeing and good health is worth maintaining as the cost of ill health, both in suffering and monetary terms, is certainly high. The analogy of only fixing something when it is broken, can be used for society's view of health. This view of health will be less acceptable in the future, as people become more informed in the areas of health promotion and disease prevention. Preventative health care will have a great influence on our health system, both in terms of availability of treatment and how it is delivered to the client. Nurses, because of their prime position in the health care system, are potentially society's principal health educators and catalyst of this transition (Lewis, 1986:663).

> *The ANF believes that the nurse provides a service which embraces the concept of total health care. The nurse has knowledge and an ability to function in a role which encompasses promotion of health and prevention of disease, restoration and maintenance of optimal health and health education empowerment of individuals to take responsibility for their own health care needs.*

(ANF, 1996).

The health of the health care system is dependant upon good public policy and government initiatives that seek to improve the health of its people as well as funding services. This line of reasoning was highlighted in 1990 when the World Health Organisation (WHO) released its findings on a study involving 32 industrialised countries. The results demonstrated that the health of the people of the United States polled very poorly, despite the country having the most technological and expensive health care system on earth (Wallach, 1997).

The WHO findings clearly demonstrate a poor correlation between money spent on health care, and the health status of individuals. Nutrition may be a modality that can complement existing health care strategies, by providing a form of preventative medicine as well as a cost effective form of treatment. Nutrition, like any other modality, will need to be evaluated in terms of its effectiveness. It should not be implemented solely based upon current trends, but rather on positive results that are cost effective to society.

For nurses wanting to gain a nutrition qualification, a list of nutrition education courses can be found in Table 8.2.

Table 8.2: Nutrition education programs available in Australia (at time of publication)

Post Graduate Diploma in
Clinical Nutrition
International Academy of Nutrition
(distance education)
PO Box 370
Manly NSW 20985
Telephone: 02 9977 0771
Fax: 02 9977 0267

Bachelor of Naturopathy, Diplomas in
Herbal Medicine and Nutrition
Australian Institute of Health Science
(distance education)
Colleges present in most capital cities
Telephone: 1800 674 717

Diplomas in Naturopathy,
Herbal Medicine and Nutrition
NSW School of Natural Medicine
220 North Boambee Road
Coffs Harbour NSW 2450
Telephone: 02 6651 1297

Diplomas in Health and Nutrition,
Certificate courses in Nutrition
Australian College of Natural Medicine
368 Elizabeth Street
Melbourne Vic. 3001
Telephone: 03 9662 9911
or
362 Water Street
Brisbane Q. 4000
Telephone: 07 3257 1883

Certificates and Diplomas in Health &
Fitness, Human Nutrition and
Medicinal Herbs
Australian Correspondence Schools
PO Box 2092
Nerang East Q. 4211
Telephone: 07 5530 4855
or
264 Swansea Road
Lilydale Vic. 3140
Telephone: 03 9736 1882

Diplomas in Nutrition and Botanical
Medicine and Bachelor of Human Health
Science (Complementary Therapies)
Endeavour College of Natural Therapies
4 Henson Street
Summerhill NSW 2130
Telephone: 02 9798 7699
or
67 Flinders Road
Woolooware NSW 2230
Telephone: 02 9544 5111

Diplomas in Iridology, Nutrition and
Herbalism
BSY Group (correspondence)
Colleges present in most capital cities.
Telephone: 1800 06459

REFERENCES

Ames B, Shigeraga M, Hagen T (1993): Oxidants, anti-oxidants and the degenerative diseases of ageing. *National Academy of Science* 90:7915-7922.

Australian Nursing Federation (1996): *Complementary and Alternative Therapies.* ANF Policy Statement:1-2.

Ballentine R (1978): *Diet and Nutrition A Holistic Approach.* Pennsylvania: Himalayan International Institute.

Buist R (1995a): *Study Guides 1, 2 & 3.* Manly: International Academy of Nutrition.

Buist R (Speaker) (1995b):The Need for Vitamin Supplementation. (Cassette). Sydney: International Academy of Nutrition.

Buist R (1997c): Preventing birth defects. *The Health Professional.* 107:1-2.

Ceriello A, Giugliano D, Quatraro A, Lefebvre P (1991):Anti-oxidants show an anti-hypertensive effect in diabetic and hypertensive subjects. *Clinical Science Journal* 81:739-742.

Davis J and Sherer K (1994): *Applied Nutrition and Diet Therapy for Nurses.* Philadelphia: WB Saunders.

Donsbach KW (1993): *Heart Disease, Stroke, Oral and Intravenous Chelation.* New York:The Rockland Corporation.

Gold S and Sherry L (1984): Hyperactivity, learning disabilities and alcohol. *Journal of Learning Disability* 17(1):3-6.

Hasse JM (1997): Diet therapy for organ transplantation, a problem based approach. *Clinical Nutrition Oral Diet Therapies* 32(4):1-18.

Harvard Medical School: Shiftwork Systems Incorporated. (http://members.tripod.com/~shiftwork) Accessed 25 September 1999.

Holmes S (1993): Building blocks. *Nursing Times 89* 21:28-31.

Kneisel C (1986): *Adult Health Nursing A Biopsychosocial Approach.* Massachusetts:Addison-Wesley Publishing Company.

Lennard-Jones J (1992): *A Positive Approach To Nutrition As Treatment.* London:The Kings Fund.

Lewis C (1986): *Nutrition and Nutritional Therapy in Nursing.* Carolina:Appleton Century Cross.

Lipski PS, Torrance A, Kelly PJ, Kames OFW (1993): A study of nutritional deficits in long stay geriatric patients. *Age and Ageing* 22:244-255.

Mahan LK and Escott-Stump S (eds) (1996): *Krause's Food, Nutrition and Diet Therapy.* Philadelphia: WB Saunders Company.

Marieb E (ed.) (1992): *Human Anatomy and Physiology.* California: The Benjamin/Cummings Publishing Company.

Matthews RT, Yang L, Browne S, Baik M, Beal MF (1998): *Neuropathology Digest-ALS.* Boston: Academy Science.

McCabe P, Ramsay L, Taylor B (1995): *Complementary therapies in relation to nursing practice in Australia.* Discussion paper 2:21-31.

Medical Nutrition Services (ed.) (1999): The phytoestrogen alternative. *Clinically Speaking.* February 1999:3.

Morley JE (1986): Wound healing. *Journal of Medicine.* 81:670.

Mion L, McDowell J, Heaney L(1994): Assessment of the elderly in the ambulatory care setting. *Nurse Practitioner Forum* 5:46-51.

Morrison S (1997): Feeding the elderly population. *Clinical Nutrition and Oral Client Therapies* 32(4):1-22.

Nurses Board of Western Australia (1998): *Guidelines for use of complementary therapies in nursing.* WA Nurses Board:1-2.

Nurses Registration Board NSW (1998): Complementary therapies in nursing practice. (http://www.health.nsw.gov.au/corporate-services/hprb/nrb-web/compleme.htm) (Dec. 1998).

Osak MP (1993): Nutrition and wound healing. *Plastic Surgical Nursing* 13:3-7.

Reilly H (1996): Nutritional assessment, identification of patients at risk of undernutrition. *British Journal of Nursing* 5(1):12-25.

Rosenberg IH, Miller JW (1992): Nutritional factors in physical and cognitive functions of elderly people. *American Journal of Clinical Nutrition* 55:1237-1243.

Stein DG, Brailowsky S, Will B (1995): *Brain Repair.* New York: Oxford University Press.

Tariot P (1994): Alzheimer disease on overview. *Alzheimer Disease and Associated Disorders* 8(2):4-11.

Teodoro B (1998): Folate, vitamin b12 and neuropsychiatric disorders. *Nutrition Review* 54(12):138.

Tierney AJ (1996): Undernutrition and elderly hospital patients, a review. *Journal of Advanced Nursing* 23(2):228-236.

Wallace E (1993): The effects of malnutrition in hospital. *British Journal of Nursing* 2(4):92-93.

Wallach J (1997): Trust Me I'm A Doctor. Paper presented on cassette. Sydney: LP Recordings.

Watson R (1994): Nutrition standards and the older adult. *Journal of Advanced Nursing* 20:205-206.

Werbach MR (ed.) (1993): *Nutritional Influences on Illness.* California: Third Line Press.

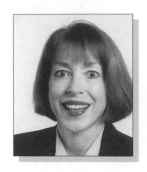

MARGARET MEYER
BA, RN, RM, Diploma of Aromatherapy,
Certificate of Massage, Certificate of Reflexology (Advanced),
Instructor in Infant Massage

Clinical Nurse Specialist, Midwifery, The Northern Hospital,
Epping, Victoria

Margaret Meyer was born and educated in Melbourne, Australia. After completing nursing and midwifery training Margaret spent six years in Britain, where she discovered and became fascinated with aromatherapy. Margaret qualified in massage in 1989, aromatherapy in 1991 and reflexology in 1996. She continues to update her professional development in complementary therapies with postgraduate studies. Margaret now divides her working time between the practice of midwifery and private practice in complementary therapies. She teaches aromatherapy and acts in an advisory capacity to health care settings. Margaret has a special concern for the implementation of complementary therapies into health care settings, and is Chair of the Complementary Therapies Special Interest Group of the Australian Nurses Federation. She served on the International Advisory Board of the UK journal *Complementary Therapies in Nursing and Midwifery* from 1995 to 1998.

Chapter 9

Aromatherapy

INTRODUCTION

Aromatherapy can be defined as the therapeutic use of plant essential oils. Aromatherapy has a variety of applications, yet it is unique amongst complementary modalities in that it uses aromas to engage the sense of smell in a healing dynamic. British surveys found it to be the fifth most popular complementary therapy after osteopathy, chiropratic, homoeopathy and acupuncture (Price, 1998). This chapter represents an introduction to aromatherapy in which essential oils and their properties, methods of application, precautions, research and case studies are discussed.

HISTORY

The use of plants for healing purposes is as old as mankind. Texts from ancient civilisations such as Egypt, India, China, Greece and Rome refer to the properties of aromatic plants. The story of the gifts of myrrh and frankincense to the Christ child suggests that they were greatly valued in Biblical times (St Matthew, 2:11). In the Middle East, the extraction of essential oils from plants evolved into the process of steam distillation in the tenth century AD. This knowledge was transported to Europe by the Crusaders in the twelfth century, and texts by physicians such as Paracelsus in the fifteenth century and Culpeper in the seventeenth century contain references to essential oils (Battaglia, 1995). In England and Europe, essential oils and herbal remedies continued to be used by apothecaries and physicians until the end of the nineteenth century.

However, aromatherapy as it is known and practised today had its beginnings in the twentieth century. The term 'aromatherapie' was first used by French chemist Rene-Maurice Gattefosse in 1937 in the title of a book in which he investigated the properties of essential oils (Gattefosse, 1993). Essential oils were successfully used in the treatment of traumatic wounds during the Indochinese war by Dr Jean Valnet, an army surgeon from 1948 to1959 (Valnet, 1980). In France, the medical use of essential oils was researched and developed by doctors such as Belaiche, Lapraz and Penoel. *L'aromatherapie exactement* (Franchomme and Penoel, 1990) is considered to be a major reference work on the pharmacology of essential oils for medical aromatherapists.

The manner in which aromatherapy is practised today in England, the USA and Australia was greatly influenced by French biochemist Marguerite Maury, who introduced the concept of using essential oils in combination with massage in the 1950s. Maury's method was initially practised in beauty therapy in the United Kingdom. The interest in aromatherapy as a modality in its own right led to the instigation of formal education for aromatherapists in the 1970s. British nurses recognised the potential of aromatherapy to enhance the care and wellbeing of their clients, and it has been implemented in a variety of health care settings in Britain. This led to formal research studies in aromatherapy by nurses in an endeavour to establish an evidence base for its use. Nurses in Australia, Canada and the United States are following Britain's example.

ESSENTIAL OILS

Essential oils can be defined as fragrant, volatile liquids which have been extracted from a single botanical source from flowers, leaves, grasses, roots, fruits, or woods. In plant life these essences impart the characteristic aroma of an individual plant and serve to attract insects and protect against herbivores. Steam distillation is the principal method of extraction of most essential oils. In the extraction process, the oils become approximately 100 times more concentrated than the plants from which they are obtained (Tisserand and Balacs, 1995), hence the need to use only small quantities (i.e. a few drops) to achieve a therapeutic effect. Essential oils are also extracted from the rinds of citrus fruits by a process known as expression.

Essential oils are often mixed in carrier oils for use on the body. Carrier oils are vegetable oils that are extracted by a process of cold pressing. Nuts and seeds are placed in a press and the heat and friction generated by the pressure forces the oils out. Some examples of carrier oils are sweet almond oil, grapeseed oil and apricot kernel oil.

ABSORPTION, METABOLISM AND EXCRETION

Essential oils are most commonly absorbed by the body through the process of olfaction. Because they are volatile, essential oil molecules pervade the air. The molecules are absorbed by the nasal mucosa which contains olfactory receptors, and are transmitted to the limbic system of the brain via the olfactory nerve, which stimulates the release of neurotransmitters such as enkephalins and endorphins. These neurotransmitters produce feelings of euphoria and decreased pain perception. Aromas have the ability to evoke memories because memory is stored in the same area of the brain associated with smell—the limbic system (Lawless, 1994). To illustrate this point, a woman whose little boy sustained severe burns was allowed by medical staff at the hospital to use lavender essential oil in the treatment of his burns. The accelerated healing rate of the burns was attributed to the use of lavender. The mother discovered that thereafter, the smell of lavender brought back memories of her son's burns (Smith, 1994).

Essential oils also enter the body through the skin. When diluted in vegetable oil and massaged into the skin they are metabolised by skin enzymes and absorbed through the pores and hair follicles into the dermal capillaries. They are transported in the circulation to the liver where further metabolism takes place, before waste products are excreted by the kidneys, and through expired air and sweat. Essential oils interact with living cells because they are known to be chemically compatible with cell membranes (Bowles, 1993). During massage, the rate of absorption of each essential oil in a blend depends upon its affinity with cellular membranes.

PROPERTIES

Essential oils possess a wide range of therapeutic properties. For example, essential oils are well known for their anti-microbial action (Franchomme and Penoel, 1990; and Williams, 1998). However, during treatment of an infection using essential oils it is inevitable that the oils will have an effect on the mind and emotions simply by virtue of their characteristic aromas. Such an holistic effect may contribute to the healing process. Imagine being confined to bed with a respiratory infection, and having the aromas of tea tree, thyme and lemon essential oils, all known for their anti-microbial action, vapourising nearby.

The difference between essential oils extracted from plants and synthetic fragrances created in a laboratory is that essential oils have a far greater range of therapeutic properties. Each essential oil is made up of several hundred chemical constituents in varying quantities (Tisserand and Balacs, 1995) and cannot be replicated by synthesised products. Synthetic oils, also known as fragrant oils, imitate the fragrance of essential oils, can smell pleasant and may have an effect on mood. Synthetic oils are not recommended for use on the body.

Practising aromatherapists select essential oils according to their botanical names because the chemical properties can be different between plant species. For example Lavender could refer to either *Lavendula angustifolia* (true lavender) or spike lavender *Lavender spica*. It is recommended that nurses using essential oils become familiar with their botanical names. The botanical names are given for the essential oils referred to in this chapter the first time they are mentioned.

SOME THERAPEUTIC PROPERTIES OF ESSENTIAL OILS AND EXAMPLES

- Essential oils are effective against a variety of micro-organisms, including bacteria, viruses, and fungi (Franchomme and Penoel, 1990). Examples include tea tree (*Melaleuca alternifolia*), thyme (*Thymus vulgaris*), eucalyptus (*Eucalyptus radiata*), cypress (*Cupressus sempervirens*), lavender (*Lavendula angustifolia*), bergamot (*Citrus bergamia*).
- Essential oils have an expectorant effect, assisting in the removal of mucus secretions from the respiratory mucosa. Examples include eucalyptus (*Eucalyptus citriodora, Eucalyptus globulus*), tea tree (*Melaleuca alternifolia*), pine (*Pinus sylvestris*), cypress (*Cupressus sempervirens*), cedar (*Cedrus atlanticus*), frankincense (*Boswellia carterii*).
- Many essential oils have antispasmodic effects that include the release of spasm and tension in voluntary and involuntary muscle. Examples include lavender (*Lavendula angustifolia*), clary sage (*Salvia sclarea*), ylang ylang (*Cananga odorata*), Roman chamomile (*Anthemis nobilis*), peppermint (*Mentha piperita*).
- Essential oils assist with wound healing by promoting granulation, reducing inflammation and inhibiting infection. Examples include lavender (*Lavendula angustifolia*), everlasting (*Helicrysum angustifolia*), frankincense (*Boswellia carterii*), myrrh (*Commiphora myrrha*).
- Essential oils have a regulating effect on the central nervous system, and their sedative effects have been demonstrated in a number of studies (Henry et al., 1994; and Buchbauer, 1991). Examples include lavender (*Lavendula angustifolia*), Roman chamomile (*Anthemis nobilis*), clary sage (*Salvia sclarea*), mandarin (*Citrus reticulata*), ylang ylang (*Cananga odorata*), geranium (*Pelargonium graveolens*).

- Essential oils with a cephalic effect are considered to be effective in stimulating mental activity. Examples include basil (*Ocimum basilicum*), peppermint (*Mentha piperita*), lemon (*Citrus limonum*), rosemary (*Rosmarinus officinalis*), thyme (*Thymus vulgaris*).

METHODS OF APPLICATION

Essential oils are used most commonly in massage treatments, inhalations, compresses, baths and vapourisers. Codes of practice for professional aromatherapists do not permit the use of essential oils orally in Australia. In Europe ingestion of essential oils is used, but only if the oils are prescribed by qualified medical aromatherapists.

MASSAGE

Essential oils are highly concentrated substances and must be diluted in a suitable carrier such as vegetable oil before being applied to the skin. Cold-pressed vegetable oils such as sweet almond or macadamia nut oil are recommended because they have a higher content of vitamins and minerals than oils which have been refined. Mineral oils are not suitable because they form a barrier on the skin and prevent the essential oils from being absorbed.

The recommended concentration is between 2% and 3%. Most commonly, 2.5% concentration is used and can be achieved by adding five drops of essential oil to 10 mls of cold-pressed vegetable oil. Lower doses are required for the frail elderly, children or in pregnancy, for example, two drops of essential oil in 10 mls of cold-pressed vegetable oil.

Massage is one of the most effective ways to apply essential oils to the body. It promotes the rate of blood flow and also raises the temperature of the skin, thus facilitating the absorption of essential oils. Massage with essential oils is a powerful therapeutic tool and promotes the release of physical and emotional tension.

COMPRESSING

A compress is made by adding two to three drops of essential oil to a bowl of water. The temperature of the water depends upon the condition being treated. Essential oils are not water soluble and float on the surface. A cloth is placed on top of the water to collect the essential oils, squeezed out, and then applied to the area being treated. Compresses are suitable for such conditions as headaches, painful joints and dysmenorrhoea. Compressing enhances the effects of the essential oils, because the oil molecules are sealed in by the cloth and prevented from evaporating, thereby ensuring maximum absorption. Absorption is further promoted by using warm water, which opens the pores of the skin.

INHALATIONS

Two drops of essential oil are added to a bowl of steaming hot (not boiling) water. A towel is placed over the recipient's head and they are instructed to inhale gently for 10 minutes. Inhalations are an invaluable way of relieving colds, flu and sinus congestion. Essential oils can also be inhaled from a tissue or pillow. **Caution must be exercised when using very hot water, and for this reason, it is safer to restrict inhalations to use by health professionals.**

Allowing a client to inhale a few drops of essential oil from a tissue is preferable from a safety point of view and allows the recipient to enjoy the benefits of the essential oils for longer than the 10 minutes usually allocated to a steam inhalation.

During inhalation, essential oil molecules pass down the trachea into the bronchi and bronchioles and may assist in the expectoration of mucus (essential oils containing cineole, for example, eucalyptus species, have an expectorant effect).

BATHS

Six to eight drops of essential oil diluted in 20 mls (one tablespoonful) of vegetable oil or full cream milk can be added to a full bath and the water agitated to disperse the blended oils. (Some essential oils such as peppermint and lemongrass (*Cymbopogon citratus*) may irritate the skin. Diluting the oils decreases this possibility). The bath temperature should be comfortably warm. Hot water can be stimulating and dehydrating.

Bathing improves hydration of the skin, making it more permeable to essential oils, and increases circulation in the dermis, which facilitates the absorption of essential oils. An aromatic bath is an effective way to assist relaxation, especially in someone who is anxious or agitated. For this purpose, oils such as lavender, bergamot and sandalwood are calming and soothing. For the relief of insomnia, a bath with relaxing oils such as lavender, orange (*Citrus aurantium*) and marjoram (*Origanum marjorana*) may be taken before bed.

VAPOURISATION

Approximately six drops of essential oil are added to water in a vapouriser. The water must be changed every four hours and fresh essential oils added due to the evaporation of the aromatic molecules. Candle and electric vapourisers are available, the latter being particularly suitable for use in areas where a naked flame would be hazardous, as is the case in most health care settings. Electric vapourisers should be thermostatically controlled to prevent the essential oils from becoming overheated and acrid.

During vapourisation the highly volatile aromatic molecules pervade the air and are known for their mood enhancing effects (Van Toller and Dodd, 1992). Vapourised essential oils are effective air fresheners and air antiseptics because they inhibit airborne micro-organisms.

RESEARCH

Although there is a lot of literature about research into aromatherapy there are relatively few quantitative studies. Most are qualitative studies. Examples of both are included in this chapter. Some authors believe that traditional research methods are too reductionist to evaluate aromatherapy adequately and that a qualitative approach is needed (Schnaubelt, 1999). Authors are suggesting that research strategies which are more compatible with the holistic nature of complementary therapies be sought (Biley and Freshwater, 1999). More information about research and complementary therapies can be found in Chapter 6.

SKIN ABSORPTION

An Austrian study measured the rate of absorption and the amount of lavender (*Lavendula angustifolia*) oil absorbed into the bloodstream following application to the skin. In this study, the lavender oil was diluted in vegetable oil and massaged into the abdominal area of a 34 year old male subject for 10 minutes. The abdomen was wiped to remove the remaining oil. Blood samples were taken before the massage (0), then 5, 10, 15, 20, 30, 45, 60, 75 and 90 minutes after the massage was completed. At five minutes traces of linalool and linalyl acetate, the main chemical constituents in lavender, were detected. They reached peak concentrations at 20 minutes and gradually decreased until baseline level was reached after 90 minutes (Jager et al., 1992).

MIDWIFERY

A study that evaluated the effectiveness of aromatherapy during childbirth was conducted with 8058 women in a large maternity teaching hospital. The study examined the role of aromatherapy in promoting maternal comfort and improving the quality of care given by midwives. Indicators used to test the effects of aromatherapy during labour were: reduction of fear and anxiety; relief of pain; assisting contractions; relief of nausea and vomiting, and improving maternal wellbeing. Aromatherapy was found to be a popular care option with mothers and midwives as was demonstrated by high effectiveness ratings. For example, the use of aromatherapy during labour appeared to reduce the need for further analgesia in a number of women (Burns et al., 1999).

WOUND HEALING

In an Australian pilot study the regenerative effects of essential oils made up into a cream for topical application were demonstrated (Guba, 1998–9:2). In Guba's study a variety of essential oils and herbal extracts with anti-inflammatory, antiseptic and regenerative properties, were combined in a compatible base cream, and given the name *Wound Heal Formula.* The formula was used on elderly patients with venous ulcers, pressure ulcers and skin tears. A significant reduction in healing time was reported (Guba, 1998–9).

BEHAVIOURAL EFFECTS

In a collaborative study, yet to be published, psychotherapy and aromatherapy were used in the treatment of children with behavioural and emotional disorders. Preliminary findings demonstrate improvements in concentration and communication, and a reduction in anxiety and agitation in three subjects aged between seven and 10 years. (Sheppard-Hanger and Stokes, 1997).

NURSING STUDIES

Reduction of anxiety
In a randomised controlled trial cardiac surgery patients in an intensive care unit were allocated to receive either foot massage with plain vegetable oil; massage with neroli

(*Citrus aurantium amara*) essential oil in a vegetable oil base; a 20-minute chat, or no treatment. The neroli blend was found to be more effective at reducing anxiety than any of the other treatments (Stevensen, 1994). Neroli contains esters which have a regulating effect upon the central nervous system.

Benefits to relatives

A study which is yet to be published examined the use of complementary therapies with relatives of critically ill patients. In this qualitative, phenomenological study, relatives were given the opportunity to give and/or receive five complementary therapies including aromatherapy. Audio-taped interviews revealed that the relatives felt calmer and were able to make a more positive contribution to the care of their loved ones in an area they had initially perceived as foreign and frightening (Brown et al., 1999).

Post-operative nausea

A control trial investigated the efficacy of inhaled peppermint essential oil as a treatment for post-operative nausea amongst patients undergoing major gynaecological surgery. The experimental group received peppermint oil (*Mentha piperita*) and the placebo group received peppermint essence. The experimental group required more analgesia and fewer anti-emetics than the placebo or control groups, suggesting that peppermint oil may improve nausea in gynaecological patients. Moreover, the cost of traditional anti-emetics was almost halved in the experimental group (Tate, 1997). In a non-nursing study, peppermint oil has been found to inhibit gastro-intestinal involuntary muscle in tissue cultures (Taylor, 1983).

APPLICATION IN NURSING

While aromatherapy may be effectively used to enhance nursing care, it is recommended that nurses receive adequate training prior to using essential oils in any context (Price and Price, 1995; Johnson, 1995; and Tiran, 1996). When using a complementary therapy with individuals whose health is compromised, nurses must be aware that they may only practise within the limits of their education and competence in that modality.

Before using aromatherapy it is important for the nurse to accurately assess whether aromatherapy is the appropriate approach to a particular patient's needs. For example, an elderly patient who is agitated may just need to go to the toilet.

SUGGESTIONS FOR THE USE OF AROMATHERAPY IN COMMON NURSING PROBLEMS

Poor peripheral circulation

Massage assists the circulation, and a hand or foot massage is particularly beneficial to elderly people whose peripheral circulation is impaired. Caution must be exercised with diabetic patients who have fragile skin and neuropathy of the extremities. During massage the limbs must be supported by pillows so the client can fully relax. Useful oils to promote circulation are a combination of lemon and sandalwood (*Santalum album*). The additional benefit of sandalwood is that it moisturises the skin.

Muscular pain

Tension in the shoulder musculature may impair the circulation and the resulting lack of oxygen to the tissues can lead to pain. The antispasmodic action of lavender oil combined with appropriate massage techniques effectively releases muscle tension and improves circulation, with consequent relief of pain. In addition, lavender is soothing and calming to the mind and has a regenerative effect upon the skin. The client is positioned leaning forward against pillows for support.

Headache

A compress to the forehead using lavender oil is calming and relieves tension headaches. The client is positioned semi-supine or seated in a chair with the head supported.

Chest congestion

Inhaling one to two drops of tea tree oil from a tissue has an expectorant and antiseptic action.

Anxiety

Essential oils such as lavender and bergamot may be combined for massage or vapourisation.

Depression

Essential oils such as orange and sandalwood may be used in massage or for vapourisation.

INFORMED CONSENT

N.B.: **When selecting essential oils for use with clients, the client's consent must be obtained prior to use.** During illness and also in pregnancy, the sense of smell is frequently heightened, and for this reason it is best to allow clients to smell the oils to ensure that they are happy with your choice.

CASE STUDIES

Ante-natal

'Susan' was admitted with placenta praevia at 32 weeks' gestation. She was ordered bed rest with toilet privileges only. She missed her family, became bored, and complained of muscular pain in her legs. After discussion with the obstetric registrar, I offered her a gentle back and leg massage with mandarin essential oil diluted in sweet almond oil, to which she readily agreed. Mandarin essential oil has antispasmodic properties and is considered to be one of the safest oils for pregnancy (Arcier, 1990). After the massage Susan said that her legs felt better and she was more relaxed. She later told me that she had slept much more soundly after the massage. I repeated the massage weekly with similar results until Susan's baby was delivered by elective caesarean section. After each massage the ward staff remarked on the delightfully relaxing aroma emerging from Susan's room.

Post-natal

'Jane', who had decided to suppress lactation, was complaining of full, hot, painful breasts. I applied compresses using peppermint essential oil in cool water to both breasts and she immediately remarked on how soothing this felt. Peppermint essential oil has cooling and analgesic properties. The following day Jane's breasts were softer, the pain had subsided, and she was able to wear a bra comfortably.

QUALITY OF ESSENTIAL OILS

When working with clients of any age it is of paramount importance to use only the best quality essential oils. Quality control of essential oils begins with the plants from which they are extracted and therefore it is important that only reliable growers are used. Essential oils are subjected to exhaustive tests by reputable suppliers to ensure that the oils are pure and have not been adulterated in any way and their chemical constituents meet the standard for the particular oil. Unfortunately, adulteration of essential oils is all too common, so it is vital that only essential oils from suppliers who maintain strict quality control are used. Reactions to adulterated essential oils include respiratory problems, headaches, nausea and rashes.

PRACTICAL ASPECTS

Purchase

Essential oils should be purchased from a reputable supplier, and not from street vendors and markets. It is preferable that essential oil labels display the common name of the essential oil (e.g. lavender), its botanical name (e.g. *Lavendula angustifolia*), the name and address of the manufacturer, an expiry date and a batch number. An expiry date is especially important with citrus oils, as they have a limited shelf life. Aust L on the label indicates that the product is listed as safe on the Australian Register of Therapeutic Goods. Aust R indicates that it is a restricted product and must be packaged in a ribbed poison bottle with a childproof cap.

Storage

Essential oils must be stored correctly to prevent oxidation and chemical degradation. They are commonly packaged in amber or dark glass bottles with a drop dispenser to enable accurate quantities to be dispensed. They must be kept tightly capped at all times, and away from direct sunlight and ultra violet light. If labelled *100% Pure Essential Oil* this confirms that the essential oil is only derived from the specified plant species. They should be kept out of the reach of children. Carrier oils must be bottled in amber or dark glass containers, and require similar conditions of storage to prevent rancidity.

EQUIPMENT

Containers

When blending essential oils with vegetable oil for massage, glass, ceramic or stainless steel containers are recommended. Plastic containers are of varying qualities and are better avoided because essential oils can react with the plastic and become contaminated. Essential oils can be blended with vegetable oil in a glass or ceramic bowl if they are to be used immediately, but if the blend is to be stored for any length of time it should be placed in an amber glass bottle and can be stored in a dark cupboard for up to three months.

Vapourisers

Electric vapourisers should be thermostatically controlled and carry a certificate of warranty. They may be purchased from essential oil suppliers. If a vapouriser is used regularly essential oils will accumulate on its surfaces, particularly very viscous oils such as patchouli (*Pogostemon patchouli*) and myrrh. Cleaning the vapouriser with methylated spirits will remove any residue.

PRECAUTIONS

- Essential oils must not be taken by mouth.
- Essential oils must be kept away from eyes and mucous membranes.

- Caution must be exercised when applying essential oils to sensitive or damaged skin, and people with known sensitivities.
- Essential oils must not be applied undiluted to the skin. They must be diluted in a suitable carrier, for example vegetable oil. Non-irritant oils such as lavender are the exception and may be used for spot application (e.g. to soothe insect bites).
- Essential oils expressed from citrus rinds (e.g. bergamot) are known to have a photosensitising action on the skin, and should not be applied to the skin for up to four hours prior to exposure to sunlight or ultra violet light.
- Inhalations using steam alone, or with the addition of eucalyptus essential oil, are contraindicated in asthmatics as they have the potential to irritate respiratory mucosa and induce coughing, which may set off an asthmatic attack (Penoel and Penoel, 1998).
- Certain essential oils are contraindicated in pregnancy because they have oestrogenic effects and may induce bleeding, especially in the first trimester. Examples include basil, clary sage, fennel (*Foeniculum vulgare*), juniper (*Juniperus communis*), peppermint, rosemary and sage (*Salvia officinalis*) (Tiran, 1996). Pregnant women should seek the advice of a professional aromatherapist before self-administering essential oils or receiving an aromatherapy treatment.
- Essential oils should not be used on babies under 12 kg (Bowles, 1995), and only in low dilution thereafter.
- Due to the strong association that smell can have with memory, great care must be taken using essential oils with patients undergoing chemotherapy, or those who feel very unwell or sensitive, as the same aroma in a later context could induce nausea, vomiting or negative emotions (Stevensen, in Rankin-Box, 1995).
- The indications and contraindications for each essential oil must be thoroughly understood.

CURRENT EDUCATION IN AROMATHERAPY

Aromatherapy professional associations such as the International Federation of Aromatherapists (IFA) and the International Society of Professional Aromatherapists (ISPA) maintain standards of education and practice. The IFA was formed in 1985 in the United Kingdom, and established its first overseas branch in Australia in 1989. The IFA standard of education is a diploma of aromatherapy that includes anatomy, physiology and massage. An IFA accredited course has pre-requisites of 100 contact hours, 300 hours of home study, 100 contact hours in anatomy and physiology, and 50 hours of recorded clinical practice in massage. Aromatherapy studies comprise 150 contact hours and 30 hours of supervised clinical practice. Participants must submit four case studies.

Graduates may then become full members of the IFA. IFA members are required to complete 10 hours of ongoing professional development per annum and show evidence of current first aid training every three years.

Many introductory course are available to people interested in aromatherapy. Lectures, workshops and home study courses are available. Aromatherapy is also taught as a component of some natural therapy courses, although the hours of training vary in length and do not constitute an aromatherapy diploma at IFA level. Information about accredited aromatherapy courses worldwide can be obtained from *www.aroma-tours.com/agora/agora.htm.*

REFERENCES

Arcier M (1990): *Aromatherapy.* London: Hamlyn.

Battaglia S (1995): *The Complete Guide to Aromatherapy.* Virginia QLD: The Perfect Potion.

Biley FC, Freshwater D (1999): Trends in nursing and midwifery research and the need for change in complementary therapy research. *Complementary Therapies in Nursing and Midwifery* 5(4):99–102.

Bowles EJ (1995): *Aromatherapy and the Use of Essential Oils.* Melbourne: Gemcraft.

Brown B, Barnes J, Clarke M, Medwin L, Hutchinson A, Macmillan K, O'Rourke G, Parkinson C, Pickering A, Roberts K (1999): Relatives' lived experience of complementary therapies in a critical care department. *Australian Journal of Critical Care Nursing* 12(4):147–153.

Burns E, Blamey C. Ersser S, Lloyd A, Barnetson L (1999): *The Use of Aromatherapy in Intrapartum Midwifery Practice.* Oxford: Oxford Centre for Health Care Research and Development.

Buchbauer G, Jirovetz L, Jager W (1991): Aromatherapy: Evidence for the sedative effects of the essential oil of lavender after inhalation. *Zeitschrift fur Naturforschung.* 46 C:1067–1072.

Franchomme P, Penoel D (1990): *L'aromatherapie exactement.* Limoges: Jallois.

Gattefosse RM (1993): *Gattefosse's Aromatherapy.* (First published in 1937. Translated from the original French text. Robert B. Tisserand (ed.). Saffron Walden: CW Daniel.

Guba R (1998-9): Wound Healing. *International Journal of Aromatherapy* 9(2):67–74.

Henry J, Rusius CW, Davies M, Veazey-French T (1994): Lavender for night sedation of people with dementia. *International Journal of Aromatherapy* 6(2):28–30.

Jager W, Buchbauer G, Jirovetz L, Fritzer M (1992): Percutaneous absorption of lavender oil from a massage oil. *Journal Society of Cosmetic Chemists* 43:49-54.

Johnson G (1995): Complementary therapies in nursing. Implications for practice using aromatherapy as an example. *Complementary Therapies in Nursing and Midwifery* 1(5):128-132.

Lawless J (1994): *Aromatherapy and the Mind.* London: Thorsons.

Penoel D & RM Penoel (1998): *Natural Home Health Care using Essential Oils.* La Drome: Osmobiose.

Price S (1998): Using essential oils in professional practice. *Complementary Therapies in Nursing and Midwifery* 4(5):144-147.

Price S, Price L (1995): *Aromatherapy for Health Professionals.* Edinburgh: Churchill Livingstone.

Rankin-Box D(ed.) (1995): *The Nurses' Handbook of Complementary Therapies.* Edinburgh: Churchill Livingstone.

Schnaubelt K (1998): *Advanced Aromatherapy.* Rochester: Healing Arts Press.

Schnaubelt K (1999): *Medical Aromatherapy.* Berkeley: Frog Ltd.

Smith R (1994): Lavender helps burned boy. *International Journal of Aromatherapy* 5(4):6-9.

Stevensen CJ (1994): The psychophysiological effects of aromatherapy massage following cardiac surgery. *Complementary Therapies in Medicine* 2:27-35.

Tate S (1997): Peppermint oil: a treatment for postoperative nausea. *Journal of Advanced Nursing* 26(3):543-549.

Tiran D (1996): *Aromatherapy in Midwifery Practice.* London: Bailliere Tindall.

Tisserand R, Balacs T (1995): *Essential Oil Safety—A Guide for Healthcare Professionals.* Edinburgh: Churchill Livingstone.

Valnet J (1980): *The Practice of Aromatherapy.* Saffron Walden: CW Daniel.

Van Toller S, Dodd GH (1992): *Fragrance: the Psychology and Biology of Perfume.* London: Chapman & Hall.

Vickers AJ (1998): Bibliometric analysis of randomized trials in complementary medicine. *Complementary Therapies in Medicine* 6(4):185-189.

Williams, LR (1998): Clonal production of tea tree oil high in terpinen-4-ol for use in formulations for the treatment of thrush. *Complementary Therapies in Nursing and Midwifery* 4(5):133-135.

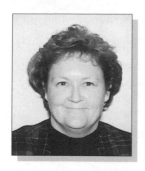

LAURIE GREALISH
RN, Graduate Diploma in Nursing (Education), Master in Nursing, Graduate Certificate in Oncology Nursing, FCN (NSW), FRCNA

Senior Lecturer in Nursing, University of Canberra, ACT

Laurie has worked in cancer nursing for many years as a clinician, manager, and academic. She is active in the Cancer Nurses Society of Australia and is a member of the Board of the International Society of Nurses in Cancer Care. Laurie's interests include patient-centered nursing approaches and how nurses demonstrate caring.

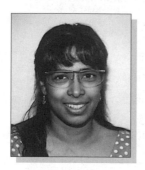

ANGELA LOMASNEY
RN, RM, Certificate in Oncology Nursing, Diploma in Therapeutic Massage

Clinical Nurse Specialist in Oncology, The Canberra Hospital, ACT

Angela has been practising in cancer nursing for 13 years. Her interest in massage stemmed from her work in palliative care at the Royal Marsden Hospital, London. She completed a course in therapeutic massage on her return to Australia. Angela has presented on the topic of foot massage at local and international meetings. Present interests include aromatherapy and therapeutic touch.

Chapter 10

Massage

INTRODUCTION

Massage is the systematic manipulation of the soft tissues of the body, particularly the muscles, tendons and skin. Massage, through touch, is one way that nurses communicate with patients. Touch is the earliest and most primitive communication tool known to human beings. Through touch, nurses can communicate an attitude of caring to patients (Barnett, 1972; and McCorkle, 1974). Massage has become an important therapy in nursing and physiotherapy.

This chapter will focus on Swedish massage, which is the simplest form of massage, and is easily learned by nurses and families. There are extensive courses in massage and a wide variety of massage therapies. Those readers interested in developing skills in other areas of massage are encouraged to investigate the many courses available.

BRIEF HISTORY OF MASSAGE

Historically, massage has been accepted as a legitimate therapy by many cultures. Hippocrates described massage as a therapeutic intervention in the early fifth century BC. Evidence of massage exists in the drawings and writings of European, Asian, and African cultures over the centuries (White, 1988).

During the Middle Ages, there was scorn for the physical body and a dearth of writing about massage in the medical literature in Europe. Some of the current popular notions of massage as 'dirty' and 'sexual' are grounded in the views adopted during this time. The notion of massage as a sexual ritual is deeply embedded in Australian culture and it may be a barrier to the use of massage as a nursing therapy. van der Riet (1995) explored the sexual nature of massage in the perceptions of nursing students and noted that they were more comfortable with terms such as 'backrub' or 'pressure care' than 'massage'. This phenomenon exists within the profession itself, with practitioners of massage preferring the names 'remedial therapist' or 'bodywork therapist' (Schubert, 1989).

Massage was revived during the Renaissance and again appeared in the literature of the time. The introduction of massage into North America in the early nineteenth century is attributed to Per Henrik Ling from Sweden. Ling promoted massage and other corrective exercises as the Swedish Movements (Schubert, 1989). Massage was one component of the three parts of the 'health spa' movement of nineteenth and early twentieth century Europe. The three components were massage, hydrotherapy, and controlled diet. As medical technology developed, massage became less valued as a therapy (Schubert, 1989) and in some areas of nursing practice, no longer exists.

DESCRIPTION

The primary intention of massage is to induce relaxation (Lockett, 1992). Nurses can use gentle massage of the back, hand, foot, shoulder, and scalp to achieve a relaxation effect in patients. There are other functions of massage, as used by physiotherapists, such as to prevent muscle contraction, muscular tension and fatigue (Balke et al., 1989) and improve lymphatic and blood circulation (Hovind and Neilson, 1974; and Kaada and Torsteinbo, 1989). The stress caused by illness and hospitalisation and the potentially dehumanising effects of the technology used to monitor and treat patients can be counterbalanced by massage, which involves caring touch and human contact (Sims, 1986).

Very little equipment is required to perform massage. The nurse needs oil or cream, towels/blankets, cushions or pillows, and a bed or table to rest the patient on. Oils, usually vegetable oils, enable the hands to glide over the skin with ease. Creams, lotions and talc can also be used. Nurses who plan to add essential oils to the base (or carrier) oil should refer to Chapter 9 where aromatherapy is discussed. Towels or blankets are used to keep the patient warm and ensure privacy. Cushions and pillows ensure patient comfort and correct positioning during the massage.

Prior to beginning massage the nurse should describe the procedure and identify the potential benefits for the patient. As with other therapies, it is essential to ensure the patient/relatives understand the rationale for performing the massage and agree to it. It is helpful to create a relaxed atmosphere in the room by ensuring a temperature of at least 20 degrees centigrade, soft lighting, and playing soft music. If aromatherapy with a candle or vapouriser is to be used, the aromatherapy guidelines should be followed. For the patient's comfort, ensure the bladder is emptied before beginning massage.

Most nurses will practise massage on patients in hospital beds or in their beds at home. A massage table is recommended for nurses who routinely visit patients at home or who are advanced practitioners, working as professional massage therapists. A made-to-measure massage table reduces the therapist's risk of back injury. Custom-made massage tables range in price from $250 to $700. Tables should be chosen based on qualities such as sturdiness, comfort for the patient, ease of setting up and carrying (light weight) and appropriate height. If more that one massage therapist uses the same massage table, the height should be adjustable.

MASSAGE STROKES

There are five strokes used in Swedish massage (White, 1988):
- effleurage — superficial or deep gliding, long, rhythmic movement to warm the muscles; the whole hand moves over the body towards the heart
- petrissage — kneading the muscle body with the fingers and thumb of each hand alternately in large C-shaped motions
- friction — focused circular movements using pads of the thumbs and fingers or the heel of hand to penetrate deeper muscle layers or work around joints
- tapotement — quick, vigorous, rhythmical strokes such as tapping, hacking, cupping, slapping, or pummelling to stimulate muscles.
- vibration — rapid shaking movements with fingers or the hand to stimulate or relax muscles.

For massage to be successful both parties should clear their minds and concentrate on pleasant sensations. Only expose the area to be massaged and keep the rest of the body covered for the duration of the massage. The technique includes first warming the oil or lotion in the hands, then begin with effleurage (see Figure 10.1). Once the tissues are warm, use light petrissage movements to manipulate surface muscles (see Figure 10.2). Medium depth petrissage is used where the large muscle masses are worked on using kneading, pulling and wringing strokes. Deep tissue strokes are achieved when the thumbs, fingertips or heels of the hands are used to reach the deep tissue below the superficial muscle layer or to work the joints. In gentle massage, tapotement and vibration are not used. At the end of the massage, the intensity of the movements is slowly decreased finishing with effleurage (Carruthers, 1992; and Ching, 1993).

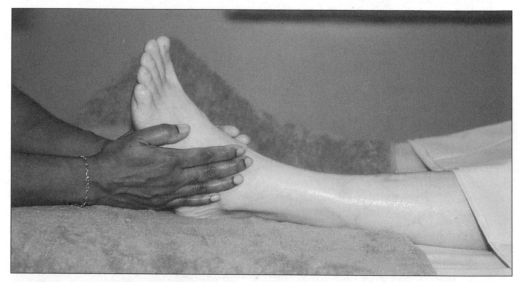

Figure 10.1: Effleurage massage strokes—long smooth strokes to warm the muscles

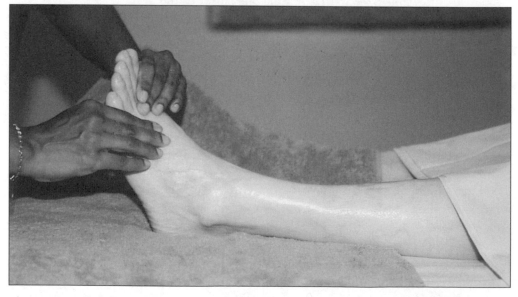

Figure 10.2: Petrissage massage strokes—light movements to manipulate the surface muscles

INDICATIONS FOR MASSAGE

The benefits of massage are described as relaxation, diminished isolation through physical contact, improved communication between practitioner and client, decreased anxiety, alleviation of fatigue, enhanced blood and lymph circulation, decreased pain; and healthy skin. In addition to people with sports and occupation injuries, populations that seem to benefit from massage include the elderly, the acutely ill, the terminally ill, pre-operative patients, the mentally ill and babies.

Massage relaxes tense muscles thereby promoting general relaxation. A relaxation response is the result of physiological changes that include a generalised decrease in sympathetic nervous activity and perhaps also an increase in parasympathetic activity. This is supported by Meek (1993) who found a modest but statistically significant effect on the physical indicators of relaxation such as blood pressure, heart rate and increased skin temperature. A relaxation effect has been reported by groups such as women with arthritis (Davies and Riches, 1995), pre-operative surgical patients (van der Riet, 1993), patients hospitalised with a diagnosis of cancer (Grealish et al., 2000, in press) and patients with mental illness (Mansfield and Blacklock, 1993).

Nurses believe that massage is important in comforting patients because of the nature of the physical contact itself (Bottorff, 1993). Working touch, like massage, can demonstrate caring and concern. Groups who may benefit from communication through touch include people with an altered body image and/or lowered self-esteem, and those who are dependent, anxious or dying (Barnett, 1972). Massage evokes an atmosphere of acceptance, respect for the body, and being cared for (Sims, 1986; and van der Riet, 1993). Nurses working with seriously ill patients in the intensive care unit use massage to convey to patients that they care for and have a rapport with them (McCorkle, 1974). The debilitated elderly, who experience physical and social isolation and sensory impairments, may benefit from the caring effect of massage (Vortherms, 1991).

When patients are touched by massage, they begin to discuss some of their concerns (Bottorff, 1993; and Corner et al., 1995). In a study in the mental health area, massage resulted in a 'release' and patients began to talk about their concerns, increasing their receptivity to counselling therapies (Mansfield and Blacklock, 1993). The close personal interaction implicit in massage strengthens the nurse–patient relationship and this in turn creates an ambience toward health and healing (Schubert, 1989).

The conversation that emerges following massage is helpful for the therapeutic nurse–patient relationship. Family members use massage as a way of communicating with each other, such as mothers massaging their babies (Booth et al., 1995), and caregivers massaging patients with a diagnosis of cancer (Ferrell et al., 1991). It is important that nurses not only use massage, but teach the techniques to family members (Byass, 1988).

Massage has a calming effect by relaxing the pre-operative patient (van der Riet, 1993). Massage seems to alleviate the fears, isolation and loneliness that can be experienced by a wide group of patients such as those who are terminally ill (Sims, 1986) and mentally ill (Mansfield and Blacklock, 1993; and Thomas, 1989). Massage can lead to enhanced feelings of self-awareness and self-acceptance. Massage is effective for the relief of fatigue. It is described as refreshing and a relief for tiredness (Bottorff, 1993; and Corner et al., 1995). Some individuals report increased energy following massage (Davies and Riches, 1995).

Massage also has physical benefits. For example, it enhances the circulation and increases venous and lymphatic flow (Schubert, 1989). It is used to benefit muscle disorders by altering blood fluidity, producing haemodilution, and therefore improving muscle perfusion (Ernst et al., 1987). It is useful in reducing lymphoedema secondary to axillary resection for cancer (Kalinowski, 1999). It has been noted that massage improves mobility and healing of the elderly following surgery (van der Riet, 1993).

There is mounting evidence to support the use of massage to reduce pain associated with surgery, cancer, and chronic conditions such as arthritis (Ferrell-Torry and Glick, 1992; Bottorff, 1993; Malkin, 1994; Corner et al., 1995; Davies and Riches, 1995; Nixon et al., 1997; and Grealish et al., 2000, in press).

In addition, massage improves the texture of the skin and skin turgor by removing dead cells from the skin surface, allowing for better functioning of sebaceous glands. Massage is helpful following the removal of a plaster cast, and has been credited with reduction of subcutaneous scar tissue (Schubert, 1989).

RESEARCH BASE

Research into massage is well developed in physiotherapy and is emerging as an important area of investigation in nursing. Areas of nursing investigation include how massage is perceived by patients, the therapeutic effects of massage, and how nurses (and lay carers) can use massage to communicate with patients.

A number of studies indicate that patients seem to find massage helpful. Corner et al., (1995) undertook a longitudinal study (eight weeks of weekly massage) to evaluate the long-term effect of back massage with and without aromatherapy. Patients reported an immediate effect that was considered very powerful and beneficial. 'Some patients experienced a sense of peace or calm, gentle soothing, "letting go" and being pampered and cared for in a special way' (Corner et al., 1995:69). Some 76% of subjects felt relaxed after the massage and 35% specifically mentioned that being able to talk to the massage therapist had a positive effect on their emotional symptoms. Most patients found massage to be overwhelmingly positive, with or without the essential oils. 'The effect of a caring and knowledgeable individual placing their hands on the body of a person who had undergone physically mutilating surgery communicated an unconditional acceptance that was deeply felt' (Corner et al., 1995:73).

Physical symptoms such as pain and anxiety have been researched qualitatively and quantitatively by a number of nurses. In a small qualitative study, using Swedish massage on five women with arthritis, Davies and Riches (1995) found patients reporting decreased pain, a sense of relaxation and increased energy. Australian researchers have demonstrated that Swedish massage reduces patients' perceptions of their post-operative pain (Nixon et al., 1997; and van der Riet, 1995). Thomas (1989) describes the results of a small study that suggests foot massage contributed to a decrease in anxiety levels for elderly patients in a psychiatric assessment ward. The authors found that pain and nausea associated with cancer decreased following a 10-minute massage of the feet (Grealish et al., 2000, in press).

Relaxation as a result of massage has been demonstrated using qualitative and quantitative methods. In a pilot study of five women undergoing radiation therapy, Sims (1986) found that massage alleviated distressing symptoms and enhanced patients' self-awareness and self-acceptance. Meek (1993) found a modest but statistically significant effect of massage on the physical indicators of relaxation such as blood pressure, heart rate and increased skin temperature. In other studies a significant improvement in relaxation following massage was demonstrated using a visual analogue scale (Ferrell-Torry and Glick, 1992; and Grealish et al., 2000, in press).

Many of the studies into massage have drawbacks. They have small sample sizes, usually less than 20, and therefore the findings cannot be applied outside the study sample (generalised). For example, in a study of nine men using back massage, there was a significant difference in pain, relaxation and anxiety as a result of massage (Ferrell-Torry and Glick,1992). A comparative trial of 21 subjects divided into two groups, one with, and one without massage, found no evidence of difference quantitatively (Fraser and Ross, 1993). Sims (1986) cautiously noted a slight but not significant decrease in subjective reports of pain in six women. Quantitative methods have been used to measure physiological indicators (signs) and visual analogue scales are increasingly being used to measure subjective experiences such as relaxation, pain, and nausea. Qualitative research methodology has been helpful in exploring massage and its meaning in contemporary society.

The effect of massage as a form of touch is attracting increasing research interest. Mulaik et al., (1991) studied patients' perceptions of how nurses use touch and found that nursing activities have changed over time to include more sophisticated assessment, teaching and counselling, and record keeping. Further, they found fewer traditional activities that provide physical comfort for patients compared with the past. They reported that most patients believed that touch meant caring and affection.

A typology of touch was developed using qualitative research methods. The typology includes 'working' touch, which involves all the types of physical contact required to complete medically related activities such as taking blood samples and changing dressings (Bottorff, 1993). In this typology, massage is classified as working touch and was described by nurses as important in comforting patients due to the nature of the physical contact itself. This view is supported by findings of a study investigating family caregivers' management of pain. The importance of 'being there' through touch emerged from caregivers' comments (Ferrell et al., 1991).

In one study, 77% of 98 patients, believed that touch conveyed control (Mulaik et al., 1991). It is not known if this group of patients viewed massage negatively. Their perception of control may be related to activities such as repositioning or turning in bed. However, the finding highlights the need for further research into patients' perceptions of the meaning of touch and massage.

EDUCATION AND REGULATION

This chapter describes a technique adapted from Swedish massage, a relatively simple therapy that can be undertaken by nurses and family members following a short lesson and some practice. Should a nurse want to practise massage professionally, a certificate, diploma or degree course in massage therapy is required. Most professional massage therapists belong to one of the following organisations:

Australian Traditional Medicine Society (ATMS)

PO Box 1027, Meadowbank NSW 2114

Association of Massage Therapists NSW Ltd (AMT)
PO Box 1248, Bondi Junction, NSW 2022

Australian Natural Therapists Association Ltd (ANTA)
PO Box 52, Sutherland NSW 2232

Membership of a professional massage association enables massage therapists to access professional indemnity insurance and be recognised by some health funds. As yet there is no mandatory registration required by the Australian government before a person can practise. There are no government guidelines for massage but each institution has their own guidelines. Most training organisations recommend at least 40 hours of instruction, including theory and practice, followed by a test before certification in Swedish massage.

APPLICATION IN NURSING: INDICATIONS AND CONTRAINDICATIONS

The use of massage in Australian nursing practice is indicated in a number of situations as described earlier. However, because touch is dependent on cultural rules and personal characteristics, such as age and gender (Carruthers, 1992), there must be attention by the nurse to individual cues regarding massage.

Individuals vary in the amount and type of touch that they find comfortable and nurses must recognise that patients need space and privacy and that touch may be contraindicated for some people on certain occasions. Patients who value their privacy may not need touch (Barnett, 1972). Mulaik et al., (1991) found that 20% of patients preferred to be touched seldom or never by nurses. It is imperative that nurses explain the procedure and seek consent before attempting massage on anyone. Permission from the client for all complementary therapies is a vital principle (Owens and Ehrenreich, 1991).

In the 1995 study by Corner et al. some patients reported feeling uncomfortable about massage for the first time and being touched by a stranger. However, these feelings did not deter the patients from taking part in the study. They subsequently reported that the intervention provided great physical and emotional benefit. These findings illustrate that recruitment of patients into massage studies requires special considerations.

Complementary therapies such as massage are used in coronary, general, pre-operative and palliative care. Nurses sometimes cite time restrictions as a barrier to implementing massage interventions. However, nurses in the 1997 study by Nixon et al. did not find Swedish massage of the hand, foot, back or scalp cumbersome. Further, anecdotal evidence is emerging in some Australian studies that nurses are finding massage useful in their personal lives (Mansfield and Blacklock, 1993; and Nixon et al., 1997).

There continues to be a powerful sexual innuendo associated with massage that can act as a barrier to implementation by nurses and patients. The notion of massage as 'dirty' or 'sexual' can lead to massage becoming a 'special secret' between nurse and patient because other nurses may view it unfavourably (Mansfield and Blacklock, 1993). van der Riet's work (1995) supports this view and suggests that nurses also 'hide' massage therapy behind words like 'backrub' and 'pressure care'. It is important for the profession to continue to challenge these values and beliefs and lead society to a greater acceptance of massage as a legitimate healing therapy. The nursing profession has established professional codes of conduct and ethics to guide nursing practice (ANCI, 1993; and ANCI 1995). Nurses using massage are challenged to describe their use of massage within the established framework of professional codes. The legal and ethical aspects of the use of complementary therapies in nursing and midwifery are discussed in Chapter 5.

As well as the cultural issues already described there are physical conditions in which massage is contraindicated:

- fractures in the area being massaged
- varicose veins, poor skin integrity, and/or skin lesions
- low platelet counts, and susceptibility to bruising
- unexplained swellings which should be diagnosed pre-massage
- unstable pregnancy, especially in the first trimester
- skin hypersensitivity such as that following chemotherapy or radiation therapy.

When introducing massage into mainstream nursing practice for a group of nurses, the nurse as change agent must first address the group's beliefs and values. Mackey (1998) discusses the valuable role of reflection in changing nursing practice to include massage. A philosophic shift is required to bring the value of holism into daily practice. Through reflection, individual nurses can compare their personal values and beliefs with each other, for example, the value of holism. There is also a need to acknowledge, and reflect on, the power relationships in the practice arena, such as the doctor's prescription of treatment (Mackey, 1998). Nurses aiming for holistic practice must continue to be reflective as they incorporate new therapies (and their inherent philosophies) into their practice.

CASE STUDY

Mr H was a 51 year old Caucasian shearer who owned a property in New South Wales. He was diagnosed with cancer of the left lung and received a course of radiotherapy but subsequently developed metastases in his bones and right kidney. His performance status was rated as '3' using the Eastern Cooperative Oncology Group (ECOG) scale. This means that Mr H was capable of limited self-care and confined to a bed or chair for more than 50% of his waking hours.

Mr H was experiencing uncontrollable generalised bone pain. When a 10-minute foot massage was first offered, he voiced some apprehension because he had never had a massage before. During this massage both his feet and all his toes were tense and rigid. Following the massage, Mr H was keen to have a regular massage as part of his nursing care.

Because Mr H had pain associated with his metastatic disease, his pain was routinely assessed and recorded using a visual analogue scale where 100mm indicates 'worst possible pain' and 0mm indicates 'no pain'. During his second massage, the nurse noted that Mr H's pain score decreased from 52 mm before the massage to 27 mm immediately following the massage.

On the third day, Mr H stated that his pain was quite bad and he was receiving Morphine and Midazolam via a syringe driver. After the massage, he remarked that he felt good and relaxed halfway through the massage.

On the fourth day, the nurse began assessing the effects of massage on relaxation by using a visual analogue scale where 0mm indicates 'very tense' and 100mm indicates 'at peace'. Before the massage, Mr H marked the scale at 20mm and following the massage, marked 53mm, indicating a more relaxed state. The nurse had further evidence of the effectiveness of the intervention.

On the fifth day of daily massage, Mr H shared some interesting comments with the nurse. He said the foot massage reminded him of his childhood. He grew up in Scotland and whenever he trod on thistles he would 'go crying' to his mother. While she pulled out the thistles using tweezers, he would fall asleep. He then asked if his wife and daughter could be taught how to perform foot massage so they could then help him when he had a bad day.

The case study illustrates a number of points:

- Mr H's initial anxiety about foot massage is common. He was keen to continue once he had experienced the massage as a 'trial'.
- Foot massage is not an onerous activity. The nurse was able to perform the massage as part of daily care.
- In this case, a 10-minute foot massage was helpful in several ways. Pain was reduced for a short time, relaxation occurred, and a sense of comfort was reported. Evidence of the effect on subjective sensations can be collected using visual analogue scales and used as part of quality audits.
- Massage can be continued as a routine therapy after discharge. Through education for his family, Mr H could continue receiving helpful massages.

REFERENCES

Australian Nursing Council (ANCI) (1993): *Code of Ethics for Nurses in Australia.* Canberra: ANCI.

Australian Nursing Council (ANCI) (1995): *Code of Professional Conduct for Nurses in Australia.* Canberra: ANCI.

Balke B, Anthony J, Wyatt F (1989): The effects of massage treatment on exercise fatigue. *Clinical Sports Medicine* 1:189–196.

Barnett K (1972): A theoretical construction of the concepts of touch as they relate to nursing. *Nursing Research* 21(2):102–110.

Booth CL, Johnson-Crowley N, Barnard KE (1985): Infant massage and exercise: worth the effort? *Maternal Child Nursing* 10:184–189.

Bottorff JL (1993): The use and meaning of touch in caring for patients with cancer. *Oncology Nursing Forum* 20(10):1531–1538.

Byass R (1988): Soothing body and soul. *Nursing Times* 84(24):39–41.

Carruthers A (1992): A force to promote bonding and wellbeing: therapeutic touch and massage. *Professional Nurse* February:297–300.

Ching M (1993): The use of touch in nursing practice. *Australian Journal of Advanced Nursing* 10(4): 4–9.

Corner J, Cawley N, Hildebrand S (1995): An evaluation of the use of massage and essential oils on the wellbeing of cancer patients. *International Journal of Palliative Nursing* 1(2):67–73.

Davies S, Riches L (1995): Healing touch? *Nursing Times* 91(25):42–43.

Ernst E, Matrai A, Magyarosy I, Liebermeister RGA, Eck M, Breu MC (1987): Massages cause changes in blood fluidity. *Physiotherapy* 73(1):43-45.

Ferrell BR, Cohen MZ, Rhiner M, Rozek A (1991): Pain as a metaphor for illness. Part II: family caregivers' management of pain. *Oncology Nursing Forum* 18(8):1315-1321.

Ferrell-Torry AT, Glick OJ (1992): The use of therapeutic massage as a nursing intervention to modify anxiety and the perception of cancer pain. *Cancer Nursing* 16(2):93-101.

Fraser J, Kerr J (1993): Psychophysiological effects of back massage on elderly institutionalised patients. *Journal of Advanced Nursing* 18:238-245.

Grealish L, Lomasney A, Whiteman B (2000): Foot massage: a nursing intervention to modify the distressing symptoms of pain and nausea in patients hospitalized with cancer. *Cancer Nursing* (In press)

Hovind H, Neilsen S L (1974): Effect of massage on blood flow in skeletal muscle. *Scandinavian Journal of Rehabilition Medicine* 6:74-77.

Kaada B, Torsteinbo O (1989): Increase of plasma beta endorphin levels in connective tissue massage. *General Pharmacology* 20:487-489.

Kalinowski BH (1999): Lymphedema. In: Yarbro CH, Frogge MH, Goodman M (eds) *Cancer Symptom Management* (2nd edn). Toronto: Jones & Bartlett, pp. 457-486.

Lockett J (1992): Reflexology–a nursing tool? *Australian Journal of Nursing* 22(1):14-15.

Mackey S (1998): Massage as a nursing intervention: using reflection to achieve change in practice. *Contemporary Nurse* 7(1):18-23.

Malkin K (1994): Use of massage in clinical practice. *British Journal of Nursing* 3(5):292-294.

Mansfield J, Blacklock E (1993): Massage: time to put touch on the agenda. Paper presented to 'Setting the Agenda', Australian College of Mental Health Nurses Inc. 19th National Convention, Sydney, New South Wales (6-9 September 1993).

McCorkle R (1974): Effects of touch on seriously ill patients. *Nursing Research* 23:125-132.

Meek SS (1993): Effects of slow stroke back massage on relaxation in hospice clients. *IMAGE: Journal of Nursing Scholarship* 25(1):17-21.

Mulaik JS, Megenity JS, Cannon RB, Chance KS, Cannella KS, Garland LM, Gilead MP (1991): Patients' perceptions of nurses' use of touch. *Western Journal of Nursing Research* 13(3):306-323.

Nixon M, Teschendorff J, Finney J, Karnilowicz, (1997): Expanding the nursing repertoire: the effect of massage on post-operative pain. *Australian Journal of Advanced Nursing* 14(3):21-26.

Owens MK, Ehrenreich D (1991): Application of non-pharmacologic methods of managing chronic pain. *Holistic Nursing Practice* 6(1):32–40.

Sims S (1986): Slow stroke back massage for cancer patients. *Nursing Times* 82(13):47–50.

Schubert M (1989): Massage perspectives in nursing. *The Lamp* April 20–21.

Thomas M (1989): Fancy footwork. *Nursing Times* 85(41):42–44.

Vortherms RC (1991): Clinically improving communication through touch. *Journal of Gerontological Nursing* 17(5):6–10.

White JA (1988): Touching with intent: therapeutic massage. *Holistic Nursing Practice* 2(3):63–67.

van der Riet P (1993): Effects of therapeutic massage on pre-operative anxiety in a rural hospital: part 2. *Australian Journal of Rural Health* 1(4):17–21.

van der Riet P (1995): Massage and sexuality in nursing. *Nursing Inquiry* 2:149–156.

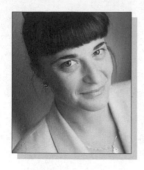

JUDY LOVAS
Master of Science, Bachelor of Arts, Diploma of Education,
Diploma of Remedial Massage

Judy Lovas developed and taught TAFE (NSW)'s Diploma in Health Science, (Massage Therapy) from 1989 to 1998. In 1998 she completed a Master of Science by researching 'The Effects of Massage Therapy on the Human Immune Response'. As a result of this study, Judy developed a keen interest in psychoneuroimmunology (PNI). She now has a consultancy based in Sydney, training health professionals about the latest research in PNI and complementary therapies and how they can be implemented in health care practice.

Chapter 11

Relaxation—the learned response

INTRODUCTION

The human body is miraculous, but it is not perfect. An 'improved model' would include a mechanism to ensure that relaxation occurs autonomically, because while the stress response occurs whenever necessary, there is no equivalent physiological or psychological response to induce relaxation. This lack of an in-built response means that relaxation must be learnt.

Relaxation techniques are vital components of nursing practice. They help reduce specific symptom distress and increase patients' confidence and sense of control. They are cost-effective, simple, and easy to teach and learn. Most importantly, assisting a patient to relax does not have to be time-consuming, it can be achieved in a matter of moments. However, success is dependent on both patients and nurses. Patients need to practise relaxation techniques regularly and nurses need to be able to teach them effectively.

There are other important considerations about using relaxation therapies in nursing and midwifery practice. Nurses and midwives who wish to incorporate relaxation techniques in the treatment of their patients must recognise the importance of their own experience of relaxation. Real insight into the benefits and difficulties of relaxation can only be gained through personal experience.

STRESS AND RELAXATION

Stress and stress response

To fully understand relaxation, it is necessary to have a comprehensive understanding of stress and its effects. The word 'stress' is widely misused. In everyday language, 'stress' is commonly used to describe negative stress, or 'distress'. Conversely, events or thoughts that stimulate, motivate and excite us result in positive stress or eustress. Without eustress, there would be no development, progress or achievement. The effects of negative stress need to be counteracted to maintain health and wellbeing.

A complete definition of negative stress includes three elements (Conduit, 1995):
- stimuli or events which are the cause of stress (stressors)
- the appraisal, perception or interpretation of the affected individual
- the undesirable response of the individual as a result of their perception of the stressor.

The following definition of negative stress includes these three elements: *Stress occurs when demands on an individual exceed their perception of their coping mechanisms and result in an interruption of homeostasis.*

The stress response equips the human body to deal with threatening situations. It is an autonomic, protective mechanism that occurs without deliberate thought or intention. The response to stress is nonspecific and any noxious stimulus or stressor may produce the same stress response (Selye, 1956). In the General Adaptation Syndrome (GAS), Hans Selye maintained that regardless of the source of biological stress upon an organism, 'the body can meet various aggressions with the same adaptive-defensive mechanism' (Selye, 1956:253). GAS develops in three stages. The first stage is the alarm reaction, which includes sympathetic nervous system arousal, adrenal medullary stimulation and the release of adrenocorticotropic hormone and cortisol. The second stage is one of resistance in which homeostatic mechanisms are engaged and there is a reduction in the sympathetic nervous system activity. Finally, exhaustion results in enlargement of lymphatic structures, an increased susceptibility to opportunistic disease, physiological and psychological exhaustion.

There are two physiological pathways for the stress response. The 'fight or flight' response occurs via the sympatho-adrenal-medullary (SAM) axis. This pathway stimulates the adrenal medulla to release adrenalin and noradrenalin, creating an immediate response by bypassing the pituitary gland. The other pathway occurs more slowly in the hypothalamic-pituitary-adrenal (HPA) axis, and involves a greater number of hormonal responses than SAM. Nevertheless, both stress response pathways result in elevated blood pressure, heart rate, glycogenolysis, respiration and vasoconstriction.

Both pathways are designed to be short-term mechanisms. The stress response prepares the body to react to immediate, extraordinary circumstances. But where the circumstances are chronic and long term, the stress response leads to conditions which may be linked to heart disease, arteriosclerosis, hypertension, arthritis and cancer.

There are two main reasons why stress today is even more dangerous to our health and wellbeing than in previous times. First, modern stressors are 'more chronic and unremitting than the episodic stressors that were typical of less complicated societies' (Lehrer and Woolfolk, 1993:10). Although war, famine and disease took their toll on the physical and psychological health of earlier societies, these stressors were essentially cyclical in nature. They were not a constant, unremitting challenge. The very nature of stress in the late twentieth and early twenty-first centuries is one of chronicity. Modern stressors such as mortgages, pollution, traffic, overwork and unemployment are constant and persistent. In this sense, the stresses upon us are greater than ever before.

Second, the constantly increasing rate of change is a major contributor to increased perceptions of stress (Holmes and Rahe, 1967; and Toffler, 1970). One of the requirements of successfully coping with life is the ability to adapt appropriately to changing demands (Lazarus and Folkman, 1984). But individuals now are required to keep adapting to a world that transforms itself more rapidly each day. 'We must move faster and faster just to maintain our places' (Lehrer and Woolfolk, 1993:11) and as the pace of life intensifies, our coping skills become less and less adequate. The chronic, unrelenting nature of stress and the rapid rate of change in modern society, then, are major causes of stress today.

Stress and psychoneuroimmunology

Psychoneuroimmunology (PNI) is a relatively new science that investigates the effects of stress on health and disease. Put simply, PNI is the science of mind–body medicine. The fundamental concept of PNI is that mental, emotional and physical health are intrinsically linked and need to be considered in relation to each other, rather than as separate entities. Health care practices can no longer be singular in their approach to the treatment of disease, or ignorant of the complex interactions between cognitive, psychological and physiological functioning.

PNI investigates the interactions between behavioural, neural and endocrine function and immune processes. Studies have shown how stress disrupts homeostasis, increases anxiety and depression and results in immunosuppression. Research into the relationship between the mind–body connection and stress have demonstrated that:

- The psychological stress of bereavement can depress lymphocyte function (Bartrop et al., 1977).
- Hospitalised patients with acute major depressive disorder have decreased lymphocyte function and decreased numbers of immunocompetent cells (Schleifer et al., 1984).
- Medical students under stress from examinations exhibit immunosuppression in response to a latent virus (Glaser et al., 1987).
- Psychological stress is associated with increased risk of acute infectious respiratory illness (Cohen et al., 1991).
- The severity of specific clinical symptoms of depression has been associated with natural killer (NK) cytotoxicity in depressed patients (Cover and Irwin, 1994).

PNI researchers have investigated the relationship between stress and immune function, and are now investigating the effects of stress management and relaxation techniques on health and wellbeing.

RELAXATION—THE LEARNED RESPONSE

Stress management and relaxation training developed out of the need to maintain homeostasis amid the rapid change and chronic stress of today's society. Relaxation counteracts stress in a non-pharmacological, non-invasive way by producing a state of physiological and psychological rest. During this state of rest there is decreased sympathetic nervous system activity.

In nursing practice, teaching patients how to relax can help reduce physical and emotional distress during all stages of disease and treatment. Specific relaxation techniques can reduce symptoms of treatment such as nausea, vomiting, pain and sleep disturbances. In the pre-treatment phase, relaxation can enable patients to cope better with fear, anxiety and uncertainty. During the post-treatment phase, concerns about the resumption of work and family life, possible susceptibility to illness or relapse and discrimination, can be eased by the regular practice of relaxation (Caudell, 1996).

However, if nurses and midwives are to effectively implement relaxation techniques in their practices, they must recognise the fundamental distinction between stress and relaxation. While the stress response is an autonomic mechanism, relaxation does not occur spontaneously. Rather, relaxation must be consciously and purposefully evoked

(Benson, 1975). Relaxation is a practical skill and like any skill, only repeated, disciplined practice will produce positive results. Success in training patients to relax, therefore, is dependent upon patients' commitment to practise. But it is also vital that nurses teach and demonstrate the techniques accurately, and then emphasise the importance of patient compliance, discipline and regular practice.

A wide range of complementary therapies may be able to encourage or even enhance relaxation. Research in PNI is now focusing on the psychological and physiological benefits of relaxation that may be gained by therapies such as aromatherapy, massage therapy, guided imagery and progressive muscle relaxation. Nurses need to remain up to date with the research, in order to inform and enhance their practice and provide patients with the best possible care.

RELAXATION—THE PHYSIOLOGICAL EFFECTS

Relaxation affects both the central and the peripheral nervous systems in the following ways:

Central nervous system:
• sympathetic nervous system activity decreases
• parasympathetic nervous system activity increases
• alpha and theta brainwaves increase.

Somatic peripheral nervous system:
• reduction of striate (skeletal) muscle tension.

Autonomic peripheral nervous system:
• reduced dilation of the pupils
• increased saliva production
• respiration slower, deeper and more diaphragmatic
• decreased heart rate
• decreased blood pressure
• increased venous return to the heart
• decreased sebaceous gland activity
• blood flow to tissues of the gastro intestinal tract (GIT) and peristalsis increases or returns to normal
• decreased stomach acidity (returns to normal)
• decreased release of adrenalin and noradrenalin
• decreased release of corticosteroids
• blood glucose decreases (caution is needed with diabetics whose blood glucose is

already low—relaxation may further reduce the level and increase the risk of hypoglycaemia)
* improved immune function.

A number of relaxation techniques can be learnt to produce these desirable outcomes. Various complementary therapies have also been demonstrated to induce the relaxation response including, acupuncture, therapeutic touch, music and massage.

RELAXATION TECHNIQUES

1. DIAPHRAGMATIC BREATHING
A lack of understanding about correct patterns of breathing is demonstrated by the usual answer to the following question: 'If you parked your car very close to the garage wall, how would you squeeze through the narrow space between the door and the wall?' The typical response is 'I'd breathe in'. This answer indicates a common and incorrect belief that during inhalation, there is a contraction of the chest and abdomen. In fact, diaphragmatic breathing causes the abdomen to expand outwardly during correct inhalation. Patients can be taught very simple exercises that will significantly improve their breathing and can be practised simultaneously with other forms of relaxation.

Benefits of diaphragmatic breathing
Increased sympathetic arousal from stress results in an increased metabolic demand for oxygen. The body cannot sustain this demand for long periods. 'Physiologically, we are like quarter horses: We can fun fast, but not for very long' (Fried, 1993:302). Stress commonly leads to hyperventilation, inability to catch the breath and frequent sighing and puffing. Deep, diaphragmatic breathing increases the oxygenation of every cell and tissue in the body and assists in the elimination of excess CO_2.

Deep diaphragmatic breathing produces a number of effects in the body.
* Circulatory system: The arterial, capillary, venous and lymphatic circulations are stimulated by the contraction of muscles involved in respiration.
* Visceral system: Contraction and expansion of the lungs and diaphragm provide an internal massage for organs including kidneys, stomach, liver, spleen and intestines. Diaphragmatic breathing stimulates renal lymph flow that is essential for healthy kidney function. It assists peristaltic movement as well as promoting intestinal circulation. Therefore, absorption of food and elimination of waste is improved.
* Respiratory system: Correct breathing encourages the disposal of carbon dioxide and

prevents a build up of metabolic wastes that assists in keeping the lungs free of bacterial diseases by increasing the flow of fresh blood.

- Central nervous system: Correct breathing encourages oxygenated blood to the CNS.
- Psychological benefits: Relaxation is encouraged by deep breathing as opposed to rapid respiration due to sympathetic stimulation. Physical and psychological relaxation are intrinsically linked via the CNS and the endocrine and immune systems.

Teaching diaphragmatic breathing

It is essential for nurses to explain the role of the diaphragm, the expansion of the lungs and the need for the abdomen to extend during breathing. During inhalation, the diaphragm contracts to allow for expansion of the lungs, while the abdomen expands anteriorly to accommodate the decreased volume of the abdominal cavity due to the flattening diaphragm. As a result, inhalation requires an expansion of the abdomen as well as the lungs. At rest, exhalation is simply the passive relaxation of the muscles used in inhalation.

The following diaphragmatic breathing exercise is simple and effective and can enhance the benefits of other forms of relaxation. Initially, the exercise should be repeated only two or three times, ensuring that each breath is as long and comfortable as possible:

- Lie on your back or sit in a chair and make yourself comfortable.
- Bring your awareness to your breath and observe it for 10 breaths.
- Place one hand on your abdomen (over the belly button).
- Place the other hand on your chest (over the breast bone).
- As you inhale, expand your abdomen first and then your chest.
- As you exhale, let your abdomen and chest sink down and relax.
- Repeat the exercise as often as is comfortable.
- Try to make your breaths long, smooth and without force
- If you feel any discomfort or dizziness, allow your breath to return to its natural rate.

Reminders for diaphragmatic breathing

- The abdomen and chest expand with each inhalation.
- The abdomen and chest relax and soften with each exhalation.
- Patients use their hands to feel the expansion and relaxation of the chest and abdomen.
- Ensure that patients' shoulders and neck are relaxed.
- Patients should never feel as if their breath is being forced.
- With practice, breathing will become deeper, smoother and longer.
- If difficulties or dizziness occur, ask the patient to allow their breath to return to its natural pattern.

2. GUIDED IMAGERY

Guided imagery, also known as creative visualisation, is a self-help technique that uses imagination, emotions and the senses to create a blueprint for what one wants in life. By means of guided imagery, a clear picture of a goal can be created, regardless of whether the goal is physical, emotional, mental or spiritual (Gawain, 1978). Both complementary and conventional medicine use guided imagery for the treatment of diseases, including cancer. Guided imagery can be used to combat stress by promoting relaxation, reducing symptoms and improving confidence and sense of control.

Using guided imagery to reduce stress exemplifies the principles of PNI, as it involves individuals' perceptions and thought processes to influence complex neurochemical, hormonal and immunological activities. Perception may also influence psychophysiological interactions since the body interprets all sensory images as real, physiological events and responds accordingly. For example, a perception of surgery as life-threatening may lead to hypertension and tachycardia prior to surgery, whereas a belief in surgery as life-saving may maintain a more relaxed and physiologically stable outlook.

Teaching guided imagery

Guided imagery is a cost-effective, easy-to-teach and flexible intervention available to nurses (Giedt, 1997). It uses a variety of devices to encourage visualisation, including pictures, aromas, and audio tapes of music, sounds of nature or verbal suggestions in a low, soothing voice. It is important to remember that guided imagery should always be a positive, enjoyable, and even fun experience for the patient. The four steps in guided imagery are shown below.

Four steps in guided imagery

1. Set your goal: Decide on something you would like to realise, create or work towards. Choose goals that are easy to believe in and possible to achieve.
2. Create a clear idea or picture: Create a mental picture of the object or situation exactly as you want it. Think of it as if it already exists.
3. Focus on it often: Bring your mental picture to mind often so that it becomes an integrated part of your life. Visualise gently, without forcing it.
4. Be positive: Create your imagery in an encouraging way.

Important considerations when using guided imagery

- Use a gentle, low, slow voice when talking a patient through an imagery.
- Ask the patient to write, record or discuss the kinds of imagery that works for them. It is necessary to determine which scenes, words, events and images are relevant and significant to the individual, rather than imposing other ideas.

- Nurses using guided imagery need to be aware of two possible outcomes:
  i) The effectiveness of relaxation can be limited by a person's fear. If negative thoughts or emotions are experienced during relaxation, it is important to allow them to occur and, preferably, for the patient to face them openly. 'Once we are willing to look fully and deeply at the source of fear, it loses its power' (Gawain, 1978:15). Relaxation may be confronting for a patient, since the symptoms of stress may be a conscious or subconscious protective mechanism that allows the person to deny deeper problems rather than dealing with them. For example, patients may find it easier to deal with the responses or symptoms of stress than to explore the more difficult and complex reasons for the stress.
  ii) Physical relaxation can occasionally result in the release of psychological tension. Therefore, when encouraging patients to use relaxation techniques, nurses must be aware of the possibility of an emotional release. Emotional responses to physical relaxation can be a frightening experience for the patient, particularly if they are unexpected. Nurses need to recognise an emotional response to relaxation and make necessary referrals for counselling.

Example of guided imagery for insomnia
- Begin by bringing all your awareness to preparing yourself for sleep. See yourself in your nightwear. Observe yourself as you go through your nightly routine. Now watch yourself drink a hot cup of milk and honey. Be aware how warm and soothing the drink is. Feel its relaxing, soothing effect on you.
- Now see yourself in bed and be aware of how comfortable you are. The room is dark and quiet, the bed linen is fresh and you have your favourite pillow. Feel how comfortable you are. Gently bring your awareness to the sensation of the warmth and heaviness of your body against the mattress and sheets. See yourself lying in bed. Focus on the position you find most comfortable.
- In your mind's eye you are still and sleepy and relaxed and comfortable. Be aware of the peaceful surroundings and the restful state you are in.
- Visualise yourself asleep. See your body in bed, resting, dreaming, sleeping. Feel how relaxed and deeply asleep you are. Be aware of your gentle, rhythmic breath. Observe yourself fast asleep.
- Now watch yourself gently wake up. Feel how refreshed and rested you are. Notice how relaxed and energised you are. Bring all your awareness to how you feel after a good night's sleep. Focus on the sensation of being refreshed and rejuvenated.

3. MEDITATION
The practice of meditation is grounded in the belief that each person has a well of inner peace at their core. Meditation is designed to enable an individual to reach this inner

peace through the practice of 'being', rather than 'doing'. Meditation can be practised in pursuit of concentration, contemplation, an altered state of consciousness, spiritual enlightenment, or relaxation. In nursing practice, meditation can be effectively used to help alleviate the following conditions:

- anxiety
- chronic fatigue
- insomnia
- chronic low-grade depression or subacute reaction depression
- pathological bereavement reactions and separation anxiety
- low self-esteem, self-confidence or excessive self-blame.

Benefits of meditation

Regularly experiencing stillness of mind, body and spirit, can enhance observable measures of health and wellbeing, such as cortisol levels and rates of metabolism. Another physiological benefit associated with meditation is a decreased rate of metabolism, even more than that associated with sleep (Benson, 1975). Meditation has also been shown to improve quality of life, even in the presence of continuing deterioration of physical health (Magarey, 1989). Studies have demonstrated that meditation can reduce anxiety and stress-related conditions (Delmonte, 1987; and MacLean et al., 1997).

TEACHING MEDITATION

Four basic conditions need to be present before a patient can begin to meditate effectively (Benson, 1975):

- a comfortable position—sitting or lying, depending on the patient's condition and preference
- a peaceful environment—a quiet, warm, well-ventilated room limits distractions
- an object to dwell upon—repeating one word or sound (silently or aloud) or looking at an object (candle or flower or photo) or focusing upon an emotion
- a non-resistant attitude—invariably, other thoughts come to mind but the patient should not worry about the content or frequency of these distractions, just calmly return to the point of focus.

EXAMPLE OF A SIMPLE MEDITATIONAL EXERCISE

- Make yourself as comfortable as possible.
- Gently close your eyes.

- Bring your attention to your breath. Take 10 deep, slow breaths, in and out, concentrating on lengthening the exhalation.
- Now as you exhale, concentrate on your word. Breathe out and say the word. Each time you exhale concentrate on the word.
- As thoughts come to mind, let them go and come back to the word as you breathe out.
- Continue for as long as you comfortably can.
- When you have finished, sit quietly for several minutes with your eyes closed. Then gently rub your hands together and place them over your eyes. Slowly open your eyes.
- Sit or lie for another few minutes with your eyes open and be aware of how you feel.

IMPORTANT CONSIDERATIONS WHEN PRACTISING AND TEACHING MEDITATION

- Diaphragmatic breathing is an excellent way to begin a meditation.
- If a patient finds it difficult to maintain the meditation, reassure them that it is not the duration that is important, but the regularity of practice.
- Reassure the patient not to worry about whether the meditation was successful or not.
- Remind the patient to maintain a non-resistant attitude.
- Remind the patient to practise regularly, once or twice a day, but not immediately after meals.

Meditation, as with all forms of relaxation, requires a dedicated approach to regular practice.

Clinical studies continue to explore the intricate relationship between relaxation and physical and psychological health.

REFERENCES

Bartrop RW, Luckhurst E, Lazarus L, Kiloh LG, Penny R (1977): Depressed lymphocyte function after bereavement. *The Lancet* 3:834–836.

Benson, H (1975): *The Relaxation Response.* New York: William Morrow and Company, Inc.

Caudell, KA (1996): Psychoneuroimmunology and innovative behavioral interventions in patients with leukemia. *Oncology Nursing Forum* 23(3):493–501.

Cohen S, Tyrrell DA, Smith AP (1991): Psychological stress and susceptibility to the common cold. *The New England Journal of Medicine* 325:606–612.

Conduit E (1995): *The Body Under Stress: Developing Skills for Keeping Healthy.* East Sussex, UK: Lawrence Erlbaum Associates Ltd.

Cover H, Irwin M (1994): Immunity and depression: insomnia, retardation, and reduction of natural killer cell activity. *Journal of Behavioural Medicine* 17(2):217-223.

Delmonte MM (1987): Personality and meditation. In: M. West (ed.): *The Physiology of Meditation.* New York: Oxford University Press.

Fried R (1993): The role of respiration in stress and stress control: toward a theory of stress as a hypoxic phenomenon. In: Lehrer PM, Woolfolk RL (eds): *Principles and Practice of Stress Management.* New York: The Guilford Press.

Gawain S (1979): *Creative Visualisation.* New York: Bantam Books

Giedt J (1997): Guided Imagery: A psychoneuroimmunological intervention in holistic nursing practice. *Journal of Holistic Nursing* 15(2):112-127.

Glaser R, Rice J, Sheridan J, Fertel R, Stout J, Speicher C, Pinsky D, Kotur M, Post A, Beck M, Kiecolt-Glaser J (1987): Stress-related immune suppression: health implications. *Brain, Behavior, and Immunity* 1:7-20.

Holmes TH, Rahe RH (1967): The social readjustment rating scale. *Journal of Psychosomatic Research* 11:213.

Lazarus RS, Folkman S (1984): *Stress, Appraisal and Coping.* New York: Springer Publishing.

Lehrer PM, Woolfolk RL (1993): *Principles and Practice of Stress Management* (2nd edn). New York: The Guildford Press.

MacLean C, Walton K, Wennegerg S, Levitsky D, Mandarino J, Waziri R, Hillis S, Schneider R (1997): Effects of the transcendental meditation program on adaptive mechanisms: changes in hormone levels and responses to stress after 4 months of practice. *Psychoneuroendocrinology* 22(4):277-95.

Magarey C (1989): Meditation and health. *Patient Management* 89-101.

Schleifer SJ, Keller SE, Meyerson AT, Raskin MJ, Davis KL, Stein M (1984): Lymphocyte function in major depressive disorder. *Archives of General Psychiatry* 41:484-486.

Selye H (1956): *The Stress of Life.* U.S.A: Longmans, Green and Co Ltd.

Toffler A (1970): *Future Shock.* London: The Bodley Head Ltd.

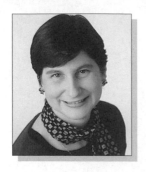

JANE HALL
RN, Midwife, Bachelor of Applied Science Advanced Nursing (Education), Master of Education, FRCNA, FACM, Member Australian College of Holistic Nurses, Therapeutic Touch Practitioner, Healing Touch Practitioner

Director: Healing Dimensions

Jane has a private practice and consultancy in healing and education. She has been interested and involved in the use of complementary therapies in nursing and midwifery since the early 1980s and was chairperson of the Nurses Board of Victoria committee which developed the first Australian guidelines for the use of complementary therapies by nurses in 1995. Jane incorporates a range of healing modalities in her practice including Therapeutic Touch and Healing Touch, pranic healing, reiki, Australian bush flower essences, guided imagery and transpersonal theory and counselling. Jane teaches Therapeutic Touch and lectures regularly at a number of universities. She also conducts seminars and workshops centered around personal/professional growth and development for nurses, midwives and other healers.

Therapeutic Touch and Healing Touch—nursing modalities for the new millennium

BACKGROUND

Therapeutic Touch (TT) and Healing Touch (HT) are healing modalities that are based on the fundamental assumption that there is a universal life energy that sustains all living organisms. Interruptions to the flow and balance of this energy are seen as resulting in impaired wellbeing and eventually illness. TT and HT belong to the group of therapies, often termed vibrational medicine or energetic based healing, where the practitioner works directly with the human energy system to restore harmony and balance (Gerber, 1988). As such, TT and HT can be placed in the company of other well known approaches to healing such as traditional Chinese medicine, Ayurveda, naturopathy and homoeopathy.

Slater (1996) further classified TT and HT as belonging to a subgroup of energetic therapies termed 'hand-mediated energetic healing' that comprises those therapies in which the hands are used as a focus to facilitate healing. Hand-mediated energy healing is a large and ever growing area and includes reflexology, acupressure, shiatsu, Qi gong, reiki, polarity therapy, kinesiology, Chiron, kinergetics, pranic healing, and spiritual healing (Bradford, 1994; Slater, 1996; Master Choa Kok Sui, 1997; Benor, 1998; and Hall, 1998). All have their roots in ancient healing practices, whether from the European, Vedic, Chinese or Japanese traditions, or indigenous healing, including those from Australian Aboriginal, Maori, American Indian and Hawaiian cultures.

However, the relationship between the multivarious hand-mediated energetic healing modalities has not yet been determined. While there may be similarities in techniques or outcomes, the underpinning philosophies, theory and practice can differ widely. Both TT and HT derive from nursing, and offer approaches that are well grounded in clinical and evidence-based practice.

HISTORY

Therapeutic Touch

TT was developed in the early 1970s by Dora Kunz, noted healer and president of the Theosophical Society in America, and Dr Dolores Krieger, Professor Emeritus of Nursing at New York University. It grew out of research on healing when Krieger and Kunz realised that the natural ability to facilitate healing using the hands exists in us all and can be developed to a therapeutic level with tuition and practice. Dolores Krieger started to teach TT as part of the master's and doctoral programs in nursing at New York University in the mid 1970s. Since then TT has been taught and used by many thousands of nurses, doctors, allied health professionals and other healers within and outside the 'mainstream' health care system. TT has become well established in the USA and is now taught and used worldwide. (Nurse Healers–Professional Associate International, Inc. (NH–PAI), 1992; Krieger, 1993, 1995, 1998; and Wager, 1996).

Healing Touch

Defined as 'an energy based therapeutic approach to healing', HT comprises a collection of energy based treatment modalities supported by a holistic philosophy of caring (Mentgen and Bulbrook, 1994:3). HT grew out of the work of nurse energetic-based healer and TT practitioner, Janet Mentgen, who developed the Healing Touch Program in 1989. The program contains a brief introduction to TT techniques developed by Janet Mentgen and interventions based on the work of healers such as Mary Jo Bulbrook, Joy Brugh, Barbara Brennan and Rosalyn Bruyere (Mentgen and Bulbrook, 1994, 1995, 1996; and Hover-Kramer, 1996). HT started as a certificate program of the American Holistic Nurses Association in 1990 and is becoming well known in the USA and worldwide.

THE THEORETICAL AND PHILOSOPHICAL BASIS OF THERAPEUTIC TOUCH AND HEALING TOUCH

A number of supporting frameworks and explanations have been presented for energetic-based healing. In essence the current literature reflects an ongoing process of melding ancient and traditional knowledge (some at least 3000 years old) with modern science. As Dr Larry Dossey (1999) recently pointed out, eminent scientists from the fields of mathematics, physics, and cognitive science have developed hypotheses that accommodate TT and HT. In the last 20 years scientists have been successful in detecting and measuring the subtle energy system, thus supporting what had previously been known solely through human experience (Oschman and Oschman, 1998, 1999). The specific theories underpinning TT and HT include: the Human Energy Field Model of Dora Kunz; electromagnetic and quantum physics; transpersonal psychology; Martha Rogers' Science of Unitary Human Beings, which relies on quantum and general systems theory, and Eastern philosophy and science (Quinn, 1984; NH–PAI, 1992; Krieger, 1993; Hover-Kramer, 1996; Mulloney and Wells-Federman, 1996; Slater, 1996; and Stouffer, 1999).

The basic assumptions underlying TT and HT are that human beings are seen as 'open, complex and pan-dimensional energy systems' comprised of the tangible physical body and an unseen, or subtle energy body (NH–PAI, 1992:1). The latter is understood as being composed of a number of energy systems or fields including energy tracts such as meridians and nadis, a series of interpenetrating vital energy fields that surround the body, and energy centres or centres of consciousness, often known by their Sanskrit name of chakras (Krieger, 1995; Hover-Kramer, 1996; and Slater, 1996). 'In a state of health life energy flows freely through the organism in a balanced and symmetrical way' (NH–PAI, 1992:1) Where there is pain, injury, distress or disease the energy flow becomes unbalanced or obstructed. Re-balancing or re-patterning the energy system enhances the inherent healing ability of the person. Life energy follows thought or intent, hence a key process in the therapeutic interaction is what Krieger (1995:13) refers to as the compassionate 'intentionality' of the healer. By intentionality, Kreiger means that both a general will to improve health and a focused goal for the healing intention are present. She describes TT as 'a mindful act based on a person's knowledge of the therapeutic functions of the human vital-energy field' (Krieger, 1995:13).

DESCRIPTION AND TREATMENT APPROACH

Equipment

TT and HT do not require any specialised equipment for practice. The client should be either lying down or seated in a comfortable chair. For some HT techniques a massage table is preferable, although not a necessity. A quiet and private space is required, however, these modalities have been used effectively in busy hospital wards and even in emergency situations by the roadside.

THERAPEUTIC TOUCH: LEARNING TO EXTEND OUR NATURAL HEALING ABILITIES

TT is a holistic therapy that works with the body, mind and spirit. The practitioner works with the client in a partnership, a healing dyad, in which both participate at a conscious and intuitive level, to re-balance the energy system. Central to the establishment of the healing partnership is the ability of the practitioner to 'centre', that is to enter a quiet, focused state of consciousness and, with a caring and compassionate focus, set their intent to promote healing for the person. The practitioner remains centred throughout the TT process which enables them to be highly attuned to the client and to accurately assess and re-balance according to the individual's needs.

Practitioners use a variety of ways to centre including using the breath, visualisation and meditation. Dolores Krieger (1998) states that remaining in a centred state is one element that differentiates TT from many other healing modalities. She says:

> ... *you are using that centering milieu as a background against which you do the techniques. In trying to form a liaison with one's higher orders of self and under the urge of passion, you can make a deeper contact with the patient which may be transpersonal in nature.*

> (Krieger, 1998:88).

Three other treatment phases take place, assessment, re-balancing and evaluation. In the assessment phase of the TT process, the client shares information about their health and wellbeing, verbally, through their general appearance and demeanour and in the form of sensory 'cues' or changes in the energy field. Cues are identified when the practitioner's hands are moved about two to six inches from the body to scan the etheric or first level of the energy field. Cues are sensory but also have a cognitive and intuitive aspect. Cues also differ between practitioners; many report sensations of heat or cold, pulsation, tingling or emptiness or fullness. For example, a person may have shared the information that they are feeling very tired or drained and have been handling a difficult situation at work. Their energy field may be found to be very close to their body and to feel very depleted except for an extended area of pressure around the head. Based on these findings the practitioner would then move to re-balance the energy field so that it feels even and smooth all over (Hall, 1998).

Re-balancing involves using the hands to clear, change or send energy. The practitioner continues to remain centred, and re-assesses the energy field as needed to guide the clearing and balancing. For instance, in the previous example, the energy around the person's head might be unruffled or cleared and the disturbed feeling calmed using symmetrical and rhythmic movements which move the energy down the body. Evaluation could reveal that the energy around the rest of the body is still depleted, so the practitioner could direct energy to the adrenal and solar plexus region (Hall, 1998).

The practitioner completes an evaluation which determines when to end the session. This is based on verbal feedback and reassessment of the energy field and involves a period of rest to maximise the benefits. In the case described in the previous paragraph, the person may report feeling relaxed and calm and their energy field will feel smooth and even to the practitioner.

In summary, TT involves four phases: centring, assessment, re-balancing and evaluation that together provide the appropriate acronym of CARE. TT takes between two and thirty minutes to perform. Less time is usually required for sick, old, frail, pregnant or small people. Babies, pets and plants require only a few minutes (Hall, 1998).

HEALING TOUCH: A KALEIDOSCOPE OF APPROACHES

HT follows a similar pattern to TT. Centring remains at the core of practice. The HT assessment process adds to that of TT to include evaluation of the energy flow through the energy centres and the remaining emotional, mental, and spiritual levels of the energy field. Re-balancing includes the use of one or more interventions selected from the HT program. TT is taught as the cornerstone for working with energy (Hutchison, 1999). The remaining technique involves placing the hands or moving them in a particular way while directing or moving energy flow through the hands. These techniques either involve the whole body or focus on specific areas. Full body techniques are particularly useful for systemic and long-standing conditions, and for toxicity, trauma or anxiety. They take longer to perform but have a more sustained effect. For instance, full body connection (FBC) is a foundation technique of HT. In FBC the practitioner's hands are placed on, or over, the key energy centres in the patient's body and limbs to clear and restore their energy system. FBC may be used on its own, or as a preliminary to other techniques, such as those used for back problems, to enhance the effectiveness (Hover-Kramer, 1996; and Mentgen and Bulbrook, 1994, 1995, 1996).

Other techniques are designed to work locally and more specifically. Mind clearing, where the fingers are placed gently on the head in various positions, is valuable for relaxing and focusing the thoughts. Mind clearing can be performed on oneself and is valuable for use after a demanding day's work. While various combinations of techniques are advised for certain conditions or situations, the final choice is based on individual assessment (Mentgen and Bulbrook, 1994, 1995, 1996; and Hover-Kramer, 1996). For instance, one client presented with a medical diagnosis of chronic fatigue syndrome. Her energetic assessment showed a picture of over energy rather than the usual pattern of depletion. The techniques chosen for her were aimed at enhancing the energy flow out of the field rather than increasing energy levels (Hall, 1999).

As with TT, evaluation is used during the healing session to ascertain progress, to select or change techniques as required and to determine when the session is completed. Full HT sessions take up to an hour or more, however, single full body techniques such as TT or localised techniques may be used where time is limited (Mentgen and Bulbrook, 1994, 1995, 1996; and Hover-Kramer, 1996).

THERAPEUTIC USE OF SELF: THE EXPERIENCE OF PRACTISING THERAPEUTIC TOUCH AND HEALING TOUCH

A major focus of the touch modalities is the therapeutic use of self as part of the healing dyad. It is therefore vitally important that practitioners are able to be reflective, honest and prepared to engage in self-development and healing at all levels. Optimal attributes are described (NH–PAI, 1992) as including:

- self-discipline
- a sense of wellbeing
- being non-judgmental
- having a holistic view of life and a sense of groundedness
- intentionality
- compassionate non-attachment and commitment to help or heal.

Paradoxically the consistent use in healing practice has been found by many practitioners to promote profound and positive effects on their own inner growth and personal development (Kreiger, 1995; and Wardell, 1999). Dolores Krieger (1998) believes this relates to the process of centring, and the accompanying healing intent and compassion which becomes part of the practitioner's whole life (Hall, 1998).

RESEARCH BASE: EVIDENCE-BASED PRACTICE

Modern research related to energy-based healing (EBH) is gathering momentum. Benor (1998) and Dossey (1997, 1999), reflecting on meta-analyses of energetic-based healing research, have pointed out the gathering evidence for its efficacy. However, as with other complementary therapies, practitioners of EBH face the challenges of studying holistic therapies within the reductionist framework of many modern research designs.

THERAPEUTIC TOUCH: RESEARCH AND PRACTICE IN TANDEM FROM THE BEGINNING

One of the great strengths of TT is that from the beginning Krieger and Kunz established a pattern of evidence-based practice. Therefore, TT has been researched consistently since the 1970s. This research basis has undoubtedly been a key factor in TT being accepted in mainstream health care. TT leads the way for nursing as a whole, being one of the most researched healing modalities in nursing. A current reference list published by Nurse Healers–Professional Associate International, Inc. (1998) cites over 60 master's theses and doctoral dissertations on TT and over 40 research based references. Overall, the research shows that of TT reduces anxiety, increases relaxation, alters pain perception, enhances and accelerates the healing process and promotes comfort particularly for the dying person (Krieger, 1993; 1997).

Specific studies demonstrate that TT:
- increases haemoglobin level
- reduces anxiety
- increases relaxation in cardiovascular, psychiatric and elderly patients
- reduces diastolic blood pressure
- reduces tension headaches
- enhances the immune response in both client and healer
- reduces stress after natural disasters
- combines well with massage to increase wellbeing and relaxation
- decreases the need for post-operative analgesia (Krieger, 1972; Heidt, 1980; Quinn, 1984; Keller and Bzdek, 1986; Quinn and Strelkauskas, 1993; Snyder et al., 1995; and Mulloney and Wells-Federmen, 1996).

In several significant randomised controlled trials TT has been shown to increase the rate of wound healing and increase the speed of callus formation after fractures (Wirth, 1990; Krieger, 1993; and Wirth et al., 1993). In terms of the classic scientific paradigm, current TT research provides what Sayre-Adams and Wright (1995:51) describe as 'preliminary proof' and even 'tentative empirical support' that TT can improve a person's health and contribute to their wellbeing. Qualitative studies such as those by Heidt (1990), Samerel (1992), and Smythe (1996) have explored the nature of TT and describe a healing relationship characterised by exchange, listening, being open and sharing experiences of calmness and peace (Hall, 1998).

Using a broad interpretation of 'evidence-based practice', indications of the effectiveness of TT also comes from reflection and review of the clinical practice and anecdotal records of many TT practitioners. By 1993 Krieger reported the experiences of over 37 000 health professionals using TT (Krieger, 1993:8). A meta-analysis of these reports indicates that TT is more effective with some body systems, organs and disorders than others. For instance, good results are recorded using TT for imbalances of the autonomic nervous system; the circulatory, lymphatic and female reproductive systems; and psychological states such as manic depression and catatonia. Schizophrenia, some collagen disorders such as lupus, and organs such as the pancreas appear much less responsive (Krieger, 1993).

HEALING TOUCH: CONTINUING THE TRADITION OF EVIDENCE-BASED PRACTICE

Practitioners of HT also emphasised the importance of research from its inception. The literature documents over 50 HT studies completed or underway. Preliminary results are encouraging and similar to those for TT (Hutchison, 1999). Healing Touch International (HTI) established a department of research that monitors and publishes updates of current activity. Studies cited by HTI during 1998 and 1999 include:
*   recovery of patients following abdominal hysterectomy (Silva, 1994)
*   pain and HT (Slater, 1995; and Darbonne and Fontenot, 1998)
*   the experience of people with cancer who use HT (Christiano, 1997; Brannon, 1997; and Moreland, 1997)
*   depression and HT (Leb, 1997)
*   HT for back injuries (Osterlund, 1998)
*   the effects of HT on agitation in people with dementia (Wang and Hermann, 1999)
*   personal transformation in HT practitioners (Geddes, 1999).

A number of case studies demonstrating the use and efficacy of HT have also been published (Scandrett-Hibdon et al., 1999; and Bulbrook, 2000).

Overall the literature reports very few side effects and indicates that the touch modalities are safe when practised by appropriately prepared practitioners working with intentionality and compassion. There are indications that the degree of effectiveness is related not only to the level of expertise, but to the personal development of the healer.

THERAPEUTIC TOUCH AND HEALING TOUCH IN CLINICAL PRACTICE

TT and HT are used in many different ways in clinical practice, ranging from a variety of private healing practices, to incorporation in nursing, medical and allied health care, in the community, in large and small health care agencies and in high-tech environments. A recent pilot project conducted in Melbourne supported the literature in demonstrating that TT (and HT) can be used effectively, even within the time-pressured environments of mainstream health care (Dawson and Hall, 1998; and Healing Connections, 1997).

From early days TT has proved popular with intensive care practitioners. In one instance a woman with Guillain-Barre syndrome was demonstrating signs of intensive care psychosis following many nights without sleep. Psychosis was averted by a TT session in the late evening after which she slept soundly all night barely waking when care and observations were carried out (Healing Connections, 1997). Cox and Hayes (1997) describe a patient who, after 87 days in ICU following a road traffic accident, received regular administration of TT. She began to sleep for up to four hours, rather than just for 15–20 minutes at a time, as she had previously. Her 'unbearable pain' ceased as did her frequent requests for opiate analgesia, and she moved from a distressed and agitated state to being able to regard those around her and the future in a more positive light.

In the area of mental health care, Gagne and Toye (1994) found that TT reduced anxiety with psychiatric in-patients and Simington and Laing (1993) showed TT reduced anxiety in elderly institutionalised people. Hill and Oliver (1993) suggest that teaching patients to use TT and visualisation can be effective in mental health. In a preliminary qualitative research project, Hughes et al. (1996) found that psychiatric adolescent in-patients responded well to TT. Wang and Hermann (1999) reported decreased agitation in people with dementia following HT, and Leb (1997) found that people undertaking psychotherapy for moderate to severe depression were less depressed after receiving HT than those in a control group who had no treatment, and the effect was still evident a month later.

TT and HT have been used effectively in pre- and post-operative care and in burns and wound care to calm post-anaesthetic restlessness, reduce pain and anxiety, and promote wound healing (Wetzel, 1993; Healing Connections, 1997; Dawson, 1998, 1999; Hall, 1998; Turner et al., 1998; and Skewes, 1999). In one case, support was provided for a person recovering from major organ transplant throughout the pre- and post-operative period with beneficial effects, including, relaxation, improved sleep and reduced anxiety and pain. The recipient felt that TT/HT strengthened and supported his own coping mechanisms and enabled him to make a smooth recovery despite his poor pre-operative condition (Hall, 1999).

Payne (1989) describes cases where TT has been used successfully in rehabilitation to assist with physical needs such as phantom limb pain, and dealing with emotional and psychological issues. In a similar vein Glanfield and Boney (1997) successfully integrated wound care and TT to treat a very angry and hostile person with diabetes who had a long-term tenacious arterial leg ulcer.

Family health is a fruitful area for the use of energetic based healing. Krieger (1998) used TT in a process which enhanced couples' relationships after childbirth. The families continued to use TT after the study finished and now second and third generations of the families use TT in everyday life. Children learn very quickly and with little tuition. Ann, aged six, received TT/HT as part of her care for asthma, and now asks her mother for healing. Recently, Ann was observed practising energy based healing on her pet (Hall, 1999). TT was used by Kramer (1990) to calm hospitalised children, by Leduc (1989) in the care of premature infants, and by Ireland (1998) to care for HIV infected children. TT has been used for women in labour to assist them handle pain and anxiety and so overcome blocks to the birthing process (Buenting, 1993; Healing Connections, 1997; Dawson, 1999; and Hall, 1999).

TT and HT have been found to be valuable in palliative care and in the care of people who are HIV positive (Newsham, 1989; Messenger and Roberts, 1994; Kreiger, 1997; Giasson and Bouchard, 1998; Ireland, 1998; and Hutchison, 1999). Families and friends can be taught to use TT and some HT techniques and so participate directly in the care of their loved ones.

TT and HT are therapies which support a person's inner ability to heal. While it has been noted that they are useful for specific conditions, and in particular areas of clinical practice, the practitioner approaches each person holistically, letting go expectations of what the outcomes might be. Physical healing may result or be enhanced, but even more significant may be the shifts in understanding of self, the surfacing of deeper pain and needs, or the deepening of meaning and purpose in life. One person with spinal injuries said the major benefit of TT/HT was 'now I feel whole again'. The feeling of wholeness enabled him to deal with the spinal surgery he needed. Another person may have physical symptoms that are related to past abuse. The symptoms may settle once the deeper trauma is recognised and healing has begun. The influence of diet, lifestyle, and human and physical environments is also taken into account and adjustments are recommended as needed (Hall, 1999).

Both TT and HT are valuable modalities for self-care and enhancing personal growth and development. One person uses TT/HT effectively as part of a process of reflecting on, and learning from, the challenges in her life as a mother, executive assistant and member of several community based committees. She has also learnt to use TT for her family. A number of health professionals have employed these modalities to help them handle the considerable challenge of providing care in the current health care system (Hall, 1999).

Many practitioners combine TT and HT with other healing modalities including medical care (Wager, 1996). For instance combining TT/HT with counselling can enhance the process of identifying and resolving deep issues. Guided imagery; the use of sound, music and colour therapy; hand-mediated energetic therapies such as acupressure, shiatsu, reiki, kinesiology, aromatherapy; and body therapies such as massage and rolfing have all been combined effectively with TT/HT. At all times the emphasis remains on the healing partnership and on strengthening and enhancing a person's ability to heal, the ongoing capacity for self-care, and available support systems.

PROFESSIONAL ORGANISATIONS AROUND THE WORLD AND IN AUSTRALIA

Since its inception TT has spread from the USA—where it is now taught and used in more than 80 colleges, universities and hospitals—throughout the world to more than 75 countries including Canada, the United Kingdom, China, Russia, New Zealand and Australia (Krieger, 1993, 1995, 1998). The Nurse Healers–Professional Associate International, Inc. (NH–PAI) is the key USA and international professional body. Some countries such as Canada and United Kingdom also have national organisations. TT has been available in Australia since the early 1980s. However, in the last five years it has become more widely known as practitioners, especially nurses and midwives, begin to use and teach it. A number of TT practitioners also offer courses for healers and the public through professional groups such as the ANF and through their own practice. TT support groups have been established in a number of states.

HT is now administered through Healing Touch International, situated in Colorado, USA. HT is practised and taught in a number of countries including the USA, Canada, New Zealand, UK, South Africa and Holland. Dr Mary Jo Bulbrook, who came from the USA to take up the position of Professor of Nursing at Edith Cowan University in Western Australia in 1991, introduced HT to Australia in 1993. HT was first taught in association with the Australian Holistic Nurses Association (now the Australian College of Holistic Nurses). Since then HT support groups have been established in most states. The Australian Foundation for Healing Touch was established in 1997 as the Australian professional body for HT.

LEARNING AND TEACHING

Core education program in TT

TT can be taught in health care agencies, or in private healing practices. There is an international certification program for TT that is conducted by the Nurse Healers–Professional Associate International, Inc. (NH–PAI). For those wishing to use TT in clinical practice the recommended preparation involves completing the TT basic or beginners level followed, after six months of regular practice, by the intermediate level course. Practitioners are then encouraged to seek mentors from among experienced TT practitioners to engage in professional dialogue and to undertake ongoing education in TT. After one or two years of regular practice, practitioners can then undertake advanced level workshops and teacher training. Plans are currently under way to establish an Australian certification process for TT. Overall, TT education reflects the modality itself in that there is sufficient structure for support but ample room for individual experience and expression.

Core education program in HT

HT education is more structured than TT. It comprises a multi-level program that allows participants to move from beginner to advanced practitioner level. Levels I and II provide the main techniques in HT and Level III offers extensive preparation for conducting a healing practice. Practitioners who have completed each level, a year of mentoring, a study program and a minimum of 100 treatment sessions can apply for international certification through Healing Touch International, Inc. In addition advanced practice workshops are available to those who have completed the basic program. Teacher training, which is by invitation only, comprises the fourth level of the program. In Australia, HT is taught through the Australian Foundation for Healing Touch. The HT program provides only a brief introduction to TT so in order to explore and access the depth and richness of TT many practitioners undertake both programs.

Ongoing education and professional support systems

TT and HT offer opportunities for ongoing education, research and professional support at state, national and international levels. Codes of conduct and ethics, and standards of practice have been developed for TT and HT together with guidelines for the development of courses and recommended scope of practice for TT (Mentgen and Bulbrook, 1996; and Nurse Healers–Professional Associate International, Inc. 1992, 1999). Monitoring and promotion of research, publication of regular newsletters, a directory of practitioners and the availability of web sites are just some of the resources available. Extensive publication of journal articles related to TT and a growing number for HT, and the increasing number of books and audiovisual materials being published, reflect the healthy state of the professional literature on both modalities.

Further education opportunities in Australia are available particularly through visits from Dolores Kreiger, Janet Mentgen and Mary Jo Bulbrook and through conferences such as those conducted by the Australian College of Holistic Nursing and Nurse Healers–Professional Associate International, Inc. Dr Mary Jo Bulbrook also offers her newly developed series of workshops on energetic healing; these represent another development of energetic-based healing techniques suitable for nursing practice.

CONCLUSION

As we enter the new millennium energetic-based healing represents the next wave of complementary therapies to become accepted and utilised by the community. Nursing has always been at the forefront to move complementary therapies into mainstream care. Dolores Krieger was ahead of her time by a quarter of a century when she offered TT at New York University under the title of 'Frontiers of Nursing' (Krieger, 1998). You are invited to share Dolores Krieger's vision of many nurses being able to use such modalities in the course of their everyday care. Both TT and HT provide wonderful opportunities for nurses and midwives to enhance and deepen their practice and their own self-care. With their sound professional structures, these modalities are tailor made for nursing practice.

REFERENCES

Benor R (1998): *Healing Research Volumes I & II.* Southfield Michigan: Vision Publications.

Bradford M (1994): *Hands-on Spiritual Healing.* Scotland: Findhorn Press.

Buenting J (1993): Human energy fields and birth: Implications for research and practice. *Advances in Nursing Science* 15(4):53–59

Bulbrook M (1998): *Energetic Healing Notebook.* Carrboro NC: North Carolina Center for Healing Touch.

Bulbrook M (2000): *Healing Stories to Inspire, Teach and Heal.* Carrboro NC: North Carolina Center for Healing Touch.

Cox C and Hayes J (1997): Reducing anxiety: The employment of Therapeutic Touch as a nursing intervention. *Complementary Therapies in Nursing and Midwifery* 3:163–167.

Dawson S (1998): The magic touch for a calm atmosphere. *Nursing Review* November: 24.

Dawson S and Hall J (1998):TT a healing modality for the 21st century. In: Gawler I (ed.): *Healing Spirit Mind and Body: 1998 Mind Immunity Health Conference Lorne.* Melbourne: Gawler Foundation, pp. 63-78.

Dossey L (1997): *Emerging Theories: Be Careful What You Pray For.* San Francisco: Harper.

Dossey L (1999): Responses to a skeptic from Larry Dossey. *Healing Touch Newsletter* 9(3):19-20.

Gagne D and Toye R (1994):The effects of Therapeutic Touch and relaxation therapy in reducing anxiety. *Archives of Psychiatric Nursing* 8(3):184-189.

Giasson M and Bouchard L (1998): Effect of Therapeutic Touch on the well being of persons with terminal cancer. *Journal of Holistic Nursing* 16(3):383-389.

Glandfield L and Boney J (1997):The healing touch. *Nursing Review* April: 6.

Gerber R (1988): *Vibrational Medicine: New Choices for Healing Ourselves.* New Mexico: Bear & Company.

Hall J (1998):Therapeutic Touch: ancient healing interpreted for modern times. *Diversity. Australian Complementary Health Association Magazine* 15:4-8.

Healing Touch International (1998): Healing touch research survey. Colorado. (unpublished).

Healing Touch International (1998): *Healing Touch Newsletter Research Edition* 8(3).

Healing Touch International (1999): *Healing Touch Newsletter Research Issue* 9(3).

Heidt P (1980): Effect of Therapeutic Touch on anxiety level of hospitalised patients. *Nursing Research* 30(1):32-37.

Heidt P (1990): Openness:A qualitative analysis of nurses' and patient's experiences of Therapeutic Touch. *Image: Journal of Nursing Scholarship* (22)3:180-186.

Hill L and Oliver N (1993):Therapeutic Touch and theory-based mental health nursing. *Journal of Psychosocial Nursing* 31(2):19-22.

Hover-Kramer D (1996): *Healing Touch:A Resource for Health Care Professionals.* New York: Delmar.

Hughes P, Meize-Grochowski R, Harris C (1996):Therapeutic Touch with adolescent psychiatric patients. *Journal of Holistic Nursing* (14)1:6-23.

Hutchison C (1999): Healing Touch:An energetic approach. *American Journal of Nursing* 99(4):43-48.

Ireland M (1998):Therapeutic Touch with HIV-infected children:A pilot study. *Journal of the Association of Nurses AIDS Care* 9(4) 68–77.

Keller E and Bzdek V (1986): Effects of Therapeutic Touch on tension headache pain. *Nursing Research* 5(2):101–105.

Kramer N (1990): Comparison of Therapeutic Touch and causal touch in stress reduction of hospitalised children. *Paediatric Nursing* 16(5):483–485.

Krieger D (1972):The response of in-vivo human haemoglobin to an active healing therapy by direct laying on of hands. *Human Dimensions* 1:12–15.

Krieger D (1993): *Accepting Your Power to Heal.* Sante Fe: Bear and Co.

Krieger D (1995): *Inner Work Book.* Sante Fe: Bear and Co.

Krieger D (1997):The inner work of Therapeutic Touch in the hospice. Paper presented to the Regional Conference of the Nurse Healers–Professional Associates, Scottsdale, Arizona, 16 May 1997.

Krieger D (1998): Interview with Bonnie Horrigan: Dolores Krieger, RN PhD Healing with Therapeutic Touch. *Alternative Therapies* 4(1):87–92.

Leb C (1997): Healing Touch research survey:The effects of Healing Touch on depression. *Healing Touch Newsletter* 8(3):15.

Leduc E (1989):The healing touch. *MCN* 14:41–43.

Master Choa Kok Sui (1997): *Miracles Through Pranic Healing* (3rd edn). Philippines: Institute for Inner Studies.

Messenger T and Roberts K (1994):The terminally ill: Serenity nursing interventions for hospice clients. *Journal of Gerontological Nursing* 20(11):17–22.

Mentgen J and Bulbrook MJ (1994): *Healing Touch Level I Notebook.* North Carolina: North Carolina Centre for Healing Touch.

Mentgen J and Bulbrook MJ (1995): *Healing Touch Level II Notebook.* North Carolina: North Carolina Centre for Healing Touch.

Mentgen J and Bulbrook MJ (1996): *Healing Touch Level III Notebook.* North Carolina: North Carolina Centre for Healing Touch.

Mulloney S and Wells-Federman C (1996):Therapeutic Touch:A healing modality. *The Journal of Cardiovascular Nursing* 10(3):27–49.

Newsham G (1989):Therapeutic touch for symptom control in persons with AIDS. *Holistic Nurse Practitioner* 3(4):45-51.

Nurse Healers–Professional Associate International, Inc. (NH–PAI) (1992): *Therapeutic Touch: Teaching Guidelines: Beginners Level Krieger/Kunz Method*. Philadelphia: Nurse Healers–Professional Associate International, Inc.

Nurse Healers–Professional Associate International, Inc. (NH–PAI) (1998): *Therapeutic Touch: Reference list 12/98*. Philadelphia: Nurse Healers–Professional Associate International, Inc.

Nurse Healers–Professional Associate International, Inc. (NH–PAI) (1999): Statement of ethics and conduct for the practice of Therapeutic Touch. *Cooperative Connection: Newsletter of the Nurse Healers–Professional Associate International, Inc.* 10(3):9.

Oschman J and Oschman N (1998): Researching mechanisms of energetic therapies *Healing Touch Newsletter* 8(3):14.

Oschman J and Oschman N (1999): How energy therapies influence tissue healing *Healing Touch Newsletter* 9(3):6–7, 10.

Payne M (1989):The use of Therapeutic Touch with rehabilitation clients. *Rehabilitation Nursing* 14(2):69–72.

Quinn J (1984):Therapeutic Touch as energy exchange:Testing the theory. *Advances in Nursing Science* 6(2):42–49.

Quinn, J and Strelkauskas A (1993): Psycho immunological effects of Therapeutic Touch on practitioners and recently bereaved recipients:A pilot study. *Advanced Nursing Science* 15(4):13–26.

Samarel N (1992):The experience of receiving Therapeutic Touch. *Journal of Advanced Nursing* 17:651–657.

Scandrett-Hibdon S, Hardy C, Mentgen J (1999): *Energetic Patterns: Healing touch case Studies.* Volume1. Colorado: Colarado Centre for Healing Touch.

Simington J and Laing G (1993): Effects of Therapeutic Touch on anxiety in the institutionalised elderly. *Clinical Nursing Research* 2:438–450.

Slater V (1996): Healing Touch. In: Micozzi M (ed.): *Fundamentals of Complementary and Alternative Medicine.* New York: Churchill Livingstone, pp.121–136.

Smythe D (1996): Healing through nursing:The lived experience of Therapeutic Touch Part One and Part Two. *Australian Journal of Holistic Nursing* 2(2):15–25 and 3(1):18–24.

Sayre-Adams J and Wright S (1995): *The Theory and Practice of Therapeutic Touch.* London: Churchill Livingstone.

Snyder M, Egan E, and Burns K (1995): Interventions for decreasing agitation behaviours in persons with dementia. *Journal of Gerontological Nursing* 21(7):34-40.

Stouffer D (1999): Why does Healing Touch work? *Healing Touch Newsletter* 9(1):3.

Turner J, Clark A, Gauthier D and Williams M (1998): The effect of Therapeutic Touch on pain and anxiety in burn patients. *Journal of Advanced Nursing* 28(1):10-20.

Wager S (1996): *A doctor's guide to Therapeutic Touch: Enhancing the Body's Energy to promote Healing.* New York: Perigee.

Wang K and Hermann C (1999): Healing Touch on agitation levels related to dementia. *Healing Touch Newsletter* 9(3):3.

Wardell D (1999): Spirituality in Healing Touch practice. *Healing Touch Newsletter* 9(3):5.

Wetzel W (1993): Healing Touch as a nursing intervention: Wound infection following caesarean birth: An anecdotal case study. *Journal of Holistic Nursing* 11(3):277-285.

Wirth D (1990): Therapeutic Touch on the healing rate of full thickness dermal wounds. *Subtle Energies* 1(1):1-20.

Wirth D, Richardson J, Eidelman W, O'Malley A (1993): Full thickness dermal wounds treated with non-contact Therapeutic Touch: A replication and extension. *Complementary Therapy Medicine* 1:127-132.

Personal communications

Dawson S (1999): Clinical case studies. Melbourne: Unpublished.

Hall J (1999): Clinical case studies. Melbourne: Unpublished.

Healing Connections (1997): Clinical case studies. Melbourne: Unpublished.

Skewes R (1999): Clinical case studies. Melbourne: Unpublished.

SOME CONTACT DETAILS AND WEBSITES

INTERNATIONAL
Therapeutic Touch: Nurse Healers–Professional Associate International, Inc. USA
http://www.therapeutic-touch.org/index.html
Healing Touch: Healing Touch International. USA
http//www.healingtouch.net

AUSTRALIA
Therapeutic Touch

South Australia
NH–PAI Australian Satellite Chapter, PO Box 98, Brighton SA 5048.

Tasmania
Therapeutic Touch Network Tasmania: Email:dixsri@bigpond.com

Victoria
Healing Dimensions: Email: janehc@ozemail.com.au
Healing Connections: Email: suedawson@optusnet.com.au
Therapeutic Touch Network of Victoria: Phone/Fax (03) 5977 5464
Geraldine Milton Email: Geraldine.Milton@Nursing.monash.edu.au

New South Wales
Therapeutic Touch Group: Email: m.nebauer@mcauley.acu.edu.au

Queensland
Therapeutic Touch Group: Email: m.nebauer@mcauley.acu.edu.au

Healing Touch
Australian Foundation for Healing Touch, PO Box 231, Mt Hawthorn WA 6016
Silversun and Co., PO Box 7055, Geelong West Vic. 3218. Telephone: (03) 5223 2203.
Email: Spiritual-Links@onaustralia.com.au

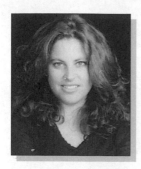

TONIA PLACK
Bachelor of Education Music Degree, Certificate of Somatic Therapy, Institute of Experiential Psychotherapy (Sydney)

I am a registered secondary school music teacher currently working as a music therapy consultant. I have produced several CDs for the health music industry. In addition to my consulting work, I have worked for the past 10 years as a somatic therapist and health practitioner in body work. Music is such a part of me that it is as natural for me to play and connect through music as it is to speak. A large part of my attraction for and affinity with music is that it can establish and harness an instant personal response and connection between people and enhance their communication. I see music, therefore, as a resource and a potentially invaluable tool that has many uses and applications.

To my mind, music is a natural source of energy within us all. Part of my quest as a music therapist is to find ways of tapping into this energy to bring about positive development. Establishing my consultancy, Essential Health Services (EHS), was the first commercial step toward this goal. It began in Vancouver, Canada, where I worked in the movie industry and created a business devoted to massage therapy sessions on location. The concept was well received and as a result led me to work in both Canada and America developing innovative ways of incorporating music therapy into people's daily lives.

Chapter 13

An introduction to music therapy

INTRODUCTION

The purpose of this chapter is to introduce the nursing and midwifery professions to the concept of music therapy (MT). It aims to widen nurses' and midwives' understanding of the origins, applications and potential benefits of MT as a form of treatment. The chapter explores the physical, emotional and environmental impact that music has on the human condition and cites research where MT has been successfully applied in a holistic approach to health care. The underlying objective is to encourage nurses and midwives to incorporate forms of MT into their work practices and every facet of their daily lives.

The chapter is divided into four sections:
- defining MT—its origins and its applications
- the physics of sound and music
- the effects of music on human psychophysiology
- making MT work for you—practical suggestions and information.

DEFINING MUSIC THERAPY—ITS ORIGINS AND ITS APPLICATIONS

What is music therapy?
MT is based on the belief that music, used creatively in a therapeutic setting, has the power to promote change, growth and development within the individual (Nordoff-

Robbins, 2000). It is a dynamic mode of treatment encapsulating a variety of different approaches including music healing, sound therapy and sound medicine. MT often accompanies other forms of medical treatment in specific areas such as palliative care and speech therapy.

The use of MT in health care is founded on the notion that 'there is scarcely a single function of the body which cannot be affected by musical tones' (Tame, 1984). The primary benefits of MT are related to:

- relaxation/stress reduction
- improved treatment tolerance
- distraction from medical procedures
- re-energising and rejuvenation
- a creative experience
- a means of self-expression
- reducing pain perception
- relieving boredom
- alleviating anxiety
- relieving treatment discomfort
- encouraging emotional shifts.

Tame(1984) reports some degree of success using MT in the treatment of:

- high blood pressure
- headaches
- asthma
- brain damage
- cancer tendency
- heart weakness
- Parkinson's disease
- Tuberculosis
- various psychological conditions, including depression, insomnia and hysteria.

MT can be applied in a variety of different ways. The MT approach chosen is largely contingent on the practitioner's orientation and skill level as well as the needs of the individual client. There are various ways MT can be implemented, adopted and utilised by health professionals. Although MT is an established mode of therapy that requires formal study, there are many ways nurses can incorporate into their work some of the underlying theory and practices of music as a therapeutic approach. MT can be applied as a self-contained treatment modality or in conjunction with other modalities.

The different forms of self-contained MT treatments include:

- listening to live or pre-recorded music
- singing, accompanied or unaccompanied, as a solo, or in a group
- creative one-to-one or group MT sessions, e.g. composing, performing, improvising
- performing in a live concert in front of an audience
- producing music recordings
- conducting
- song writing.

Music can be successfully integrated with other health practices and modalities. It is extremely beneficial combined with expressive art therapies, gentle movement, visualisation and guided imagery, natural medicines, body work, massage, energetic therapies, yoga, exercise, meditation and other relaxation techniques.

HISTORY OF MUSIC THERAPY

Music in ancient times was believed to be able to renew the divine harmony and rhythm of a person's body, emotions and mind. All forms of sickness and disease (mental or physical) were regarded as being problems able to be cured or alleviated through music. For example, it was often thought that a person became sick as a result of losing their 'inner harmony' and being 'out of tune' with the universe and its laws. Audible music was therefore used to realign the patient with the universe they lived in. The ability to create altered states of consciousness through drumming, chanting and music is probably as old as music itself. Tibetan bells, or Ting Shaís, have been used in Buddhist meditation practice for many centuries.

From their surviving writings, we know that music was used as a therapeutic tool by ancient societies including the Hindus and the Greeks. There is little doubt that ancient healers and philosophers viewed music as a bridge between body, mind, soul and the earth (Campbell, 1991). The first book of Samuel (1:16 verse 28) describes how David freed Saul of an obsessive depression through music. Hippocrates, the 'father of medicine' is said to have taken his patients suffering from mental illness to the Temple of Aesculapius to listen to the stirring music there.

In ancient China only certain rhythms, melodies and modes were deemed to be correct and beneficial. In India it was believed that there would be a natural disaster if music were played incorrectly. The Arabs of the thirteenth century had music rooms in their hospitals. Paracelsus practised what he called 'musical medicine'. He used specific compositions for specific mental, moral and physical maladies.

Medieval physicians often used minstrels to play for convalescing patients, thus speeding their recovery. Even from the latter years of the nineteenth century we have reports of an orchestra being used to treat nervous cases in a curative capacity. Mozart, a Freemason, held firmly to the Masonic belief that art was an instrument that should be used for the elevation and freedom of humanity (Tame, 1984).

It has been recognised over the centuries that the strength of music is that it works on multiple dimensions in impacting the human condition. It is interesting that as we enter the new millennium a more holistic and multifaceted approach to health care encompassing complementary therapies is becoming increasingly popular in the general community. Today, healers and therapists working with sound and music have the potential to follow in the paths of the ancient healing traditions, combining magic and mysticism with modern science and technology.

MT has been of particular interest to medical researchers and practitioners over the past two decades (Davis and Gfeller, 1992; Ellis and Brighthouse, 1952; and Curtis, 1986). The primary area of interest has been music and its effects on how change occurs in a client somatically, emotionally and cognitively.

The amount of nursing research into music therapy has increased significantly, with over 170 records published in the last five years. There are certainly many studies that confirm the ability of music to reduce pain and anxiety (for example Albert, 1996; Wiand, 1997; Trauger-Querry and Haghighi, 1999; and White, 1999), but some other interesting effects have also been discovered.

THE PHYSICS OF SOUND AND MUSIC

Music is a force that affects all those who hear it.
> *It creates order out of chaos: for rhythm imposes unanimity upon the divergent, melody imposes continuity upon the disjointed, and harmony imposes compatibility upon the incongruous.*
>
> (Menuhuin, 1972).

The human body is driven by its own rhythms. Our heart rate, respiration and brain waves all entrain to each other. Slow down your breath, for example, and you slow your heart beat and brain waves. Conversely, if you are able to slow down your heartbeat and brain waves you can affect your heart rate and respiration. This is one of the key principles of biofeedback (Campbell, 1991).

THE EFFECT OF MUSIC ON HUMAN PSYCHOPHYSIOLOGY

Music has the power to hold attention, challenge the intellect and modify one's emotional state. It can demand a moment-by-moment involvement of individuals, altering their perception of time and reducing the suffering resulting from the sensation of pain (Brown et al., 1989).

Research has demonstrated the variable effect of music on human physiological behaviour (Benenzon, 1993). Muscular energy decreases or increases depending on the rhythm of different types of music being listened to. The rate of breathing and body fatigue has been shown to accelerate or change its regularity in response to different music. Benenzon also found the possibility of a marked but variable effect on heart rate, blood pressure and endocrine function, and observed changes in metabolism and biosynthesis of various enzymatic processes. In another study Ellis and Brighthouse (1952) found that the body's respiration rate can be significantly affected by music. They found that listening to rhythmically stimulating music increased the rate of respiration.

When the tempo of the music is heard or felt at the same or a slower rate than the regular heart beat, it is said to have more of a calming effect than a fast tempo, which has a provocative effect. The average heart rate is between 65 and 80 beats per minute. However, two individual responses to the same tempo are known to occur, thus the response to the rate of the musical beats needs to be considered on an individual basis.

POSITIVE EFFECTS

We are consistently affected by music and sounds that are within our audible range. Over 80% of our body mass is actually water which resonates to sound. Research has found that there is scarcely a single function of the body that cannot be affected by musical tones. The type of physical effects music has on the body and mind include:
*   speeding or slowing, regularising or irregularising heartbeat
*   relaxing or jarring the nerves
*   elevating or lowering blood pressure
*   improving digestion
*   changing the rate of respiration
*   changing and/or enhancing the emotional state
*   influencing our desires
*   improving intellectual functioning.

Bone marrow transplant patients receiving high doses of chemotherapy found to experience less nausea and fewer episodes of vomiting when music was used as a diversion (Ezzone et al., 1998). An interesting study involving premature babies found that multimodal stimulation and singing of *Brahm's Lullaby* decreased length of stay in hospital in females and increased weight gain in both male and female babies (Standley, 1998). Children being immunised showed significantly decreased distress scores when lullabies were played (Megel et al., 1998).

The frequency and volatility of aggressive behaviour in people with dementia was decreased when patients could listen to their preferred music during caregiving (Clark et al., 1998). Music has also been found to improve mood states in depressed women (Lai, 1999), and it can be used to facilitate communication and engage the spiritual dimension of those in the care of nurses (Updike, 1998; and Brewer, 1998).

Investigations have shown that music affects digestion, internal secretions, circulation, nutrition, metabolism and respiration. Even the neural networks of the brain have been found to be sensitive to harmonic principles. Some interesting effects of music have been described including studies supporting the possibility that listening to one's favourite music causes endorphins to be released into the bloodstream. It is interesting to note that the roots of the auditory nerves are more widely distributed and possess more extensive connections than those of any other nerves in the body (Podolsky, 1945).

Music may alter components of the total pain experience and thus diminish the perception of pain. Therefore, music can be offered as a distraction, to reduce anxiety, to aid in relaxation, or as a vehicle for supportive psychotherapy. Further, music can engage, activate and alter affective, cognitive and sensory processes through distraction, alteration of mood and improved sense of control.

NEGATIVE REACTIONS

Given the dynamic nature of music, it affects individuals in varying ways. Some approaches are useful and some can cause negative reactions in clients. For example, music can enhance an individual's perception of pain therefore some caution should be taken when deciding which type of therapeutic approach will be used.

Music needs to be used and offered in a sensitive way. An example of a negative reaction to music includes musicogenic epilepsy, a rare condition in which music directly triggers an epileptic seizure. More often, a person has an adverse reaction to a particular style of music, the way it is played or the sound quality of the music being listened to. This reaction may result in increased stress and discomfort and actually reduce the healing effects of music.

In addition, the volume level at which the music is played can be detrimental to the use of music. Ambient sound levels in a psychiatric setting were found to peak between 85 and 90 decibels (DB), a range that can cause physiological stress and hearing loss (Holmberg and Coon, 1999). These authors suggested that such sound stress may negatively influence behaviour in patients with acute psychiatric symptoms.

When music is played at a lower volume, it is more likely to support the atmosphere rather than provoking it or adding another form of distraction. Even to play music that has a continuous flowing feel at a low volume, so that it is almost inaudible, can be very effective, particularly when there are already many other sounds and noises being heard, such as workplace sounds. Music at a low level can be played for a long time and can subtly engender calmness in an environment.

Other factors that may influence the client's reaction (positive or negative) include:
• the time and place of experiencing music
• the consensus required when music is played publicly
• the instrumentation chosen, i.e. natural or synthesised
• music with or without words
• preferences for familiar or unfamiliar music
• electronic or acoustic recording
• the length of the piece of music played
• the attention span and energy levels of the client.

Statton and Zalanowski (1984) found that no particular type of music was more helpful than any other in relaxation training. They found that some patients prefer to relax to well known music, while others prefer to listen to music without any known associations for them. Surprisingly some people relaxed and showed signs of reduced pain when listening to fast, loud, syncopated dance music.

It is evident that there can be completely different reactions to the same piece of music. Thus there is no conclusive way of implementing MT without incorporating individual tastes and specific needs. One of the core skills of the music therapist is to be sensitive to these needs and identify the style and mode of MT techniques that will have the greatest impact.

THERAPEUTIC APPLICATIONS

Singing phrases or instructions may help communication with patients who have oral communicative conditions such as stuttering. Communicative singing has been found to be highly effective in encouraging the development of verbal retention and to broaden patients' phrasing, possibly leading to the capacity for longer sentences. For example, sing the phrase with a rhythm and a tune: 'Do you want to go to the toilet?' Singing a question encourages a sung response and it can also be relaxing and provides an opening for the caregiver to sing-speak sentences.

There have been major advances in the use and adaptation of musical instruments to assist the handicapped (Baily, 1973; and Peggie, 1981). Occupational therapists and music therapists frequently use musical instruments as a tool to assist patient rehabilitation. Spintge (1993) describes the use of anxiolytic music in medical and surgical procedures to reduce stress, anxiety, and pain. From a psychological point of view, Spintge reported significantly reduced anxiety and improved compliance, particularly during the preparation phases before surgical procedures. The physiological measurements he recorded indicated that patients required significantly reduced amounts of medication for pain management during surgery.

It is often said that music taps into the memory, bringing to the surface many deeply buried emotional issues and past experiences. Therefore, it is often used by psychotherapists and psychiatrists as an effective tool to encourage the patient or client to reveal aspects of their past not easily revealed through general dialogue. It is also used by these practitioners to reduce emotional stress or relieve anxiety by replaying specific music that has positive associations or memories for the client.

There are many music therapists who specialise in palliative care. These therapists use music in the last days of the patient's life as a primary means of support and pain release and to reduce the fear of death. Moreover, music is used to allow the patient to communicate last wishes or an understanding of past experiences. Interestingly, Lloyd-Green (1998) found that songs written by palliative care patients in music therapy sessions expressed themes such as:
- messages
- self-reflections
- compliments
- memories
- reflections upon significant others, including pets
- self-expression of adversity

- imagery
- prayers.

MAKING MUSIC THERAPY WORK FOR YOU: PRACTICAL SUGGESTIONS

Equipment required

The equipment used in MT depends on its application and implementation. Commonly used tools in making and listening to music include:

- stand-alone hi-fi systems
- portable CD players with headphones and/or portable speakers
- public address systems
- car stereo systems
- microphones and amplifiers
- tape recorders
- dictaphones
- personal computer CD-Rom drives
- musical instruments, including keyboards, guitar, woodwind, percussion and other portable instruments.

Music systems vary enormously in cost and size. Having the appropriate system for the required space is important. It may be appropriate to use piped music linked to one control panel, a portable music player, or CD players with headphones. Headphones can be very effective for specific patients, to complement their prescribed health treatment, and as an effective tool for staff as a means of stress management.

One specific idea is to use split or double headphone jacks enabling two (or more) headphones to be plugged in at one time. This arrangement allows specific groups of patients/clients to be involved in an MT session without disturbing those around them. It is a very inexpensive option and can be lots of fun.

Suggested strategies

One way to implement MT in the workplace includes establishing a special retreat, music room or 'healing space' in or near the nursing areas. This space should have a comforting visual atmosphere, relaxed seating arrangements and a variety of playing and listening equipment as discussed previously.

Other, slightly less elaborate options include:

- instituting a relaxation music hour in the ward
- promoting BYO music

- playing music at a low level, setting the atmosphere
- having music playing continuously (using the 'repeat' button) so music is on before you enter the space.

Another option to consider is inviting a qualified MT therapist to provide individual sessions or ongoing courses, or to be a consultant or in-house trainer. You could also seek to put MT techniques and practices on the regular staff meeting agenda and communicate and share ideas about how it may be applied most effectively.

SELECTING APPROPRIATE MUSIC

When playing music publicly there needs to be consensus about the music being played. One good approach can be to hand out a survey on choices of music that can also be a means of raising awareness about preferred musical styles. Personal taste can also be affected by the instrumentation of the music. It is not an easy task to refer to music that I may find to be beautiful, inspiring and healing. We all have our own tastes and reactions. My father relaxes to *Brahms Concertos*, I find them to be stimulating and sometimes muscle tensing. If I were to create a list there would hundreds and hundreds of recordings I would need to refer to.

We all have our own personal preferences and tastes, whether they are synthesised sounds or nature sounds. Becoming more aware of your responses and reactions to differing styles of music, to the form of music and how you hear it can increase the positive effects that music can create. A list of some of the different styles of music is shown in Table 13.1.

It should be noted that royalty payments may apply when performing or playing copyright music in a public area. Fees are usually exempted for wards, consulting rooms and any area where people are sleeping. Please contact the Australian Performing Rights Association for further information. Their internet address is *www.apra.com.au*

WAYS TO STUDY MUSIC THERAPY

Music therapy, like other forms of health care, has both conventional and alternative forms of education. Undergraduate and postgraduate award courses in MT are offered by leading tertiary institutions in Australia including the University of Melbourne (*www.unimelb.edu.au*), the University of Queensland (*www.uoq.edu.au*), the

Table 13.1: Differing styles of music presented alphabetically

Acoustic	Glam	Opera
African	Gospel	Popular
Ambient/Atmospheric	Gothic	Psychedelic rock
Baroque	Gregorian chant	Punk
Big beat	Grunge	R&B
Blue grass	Health music	Rap
Blues Cajun	Heavy metal	Reggae
Chamber music	Hip hop	Reminiscing
Chilling out	House	Rock
Choral	Indigenous	Rock'n'roll
Classic	Industrial	Rockabilly
Classical	Inspirational/Creative	Romancing
Country and Western	Instrumental	Shagging
Dance	Jazz	Sing-a-long
Disco	Latin	Soul
Driving/Cruising	Melancholy	Sound scape
Early music	Modern rock	Surf
Flamenco	Music hall	Thinking
Folk	Muzak	Trance
Funk	New age	Trip hop
Getting psyched	New wave	World

University of Technology, Sydney (*www.uts.edu.au*) and the University of Western Sydney (Nepean) Nordoff-Robbins Music Therapy Centre (*www.uws.edu.au*). Please note that many of these courses require students to be proficient musicians prior to entry. The best way to access information on these courses is through the Australian Music Therapy Association (AMTA) (*www.austmta.org.au*). AMTA will only register graduates of these four institutions as Music Therapists.

There is a vast array of short and non-award courses in MT in Australia and overseas, particularly in Europe and North America. These courses cover a variety of topics and styles of MT including sound therapy, sound and vibration studies, toning, vibrational healing, natural voice movement, music thanatology (music for the dying), creative music therapy, music for healing, and many others. The best way to access information on these courses is on the internet.

CONCLUSION

This chapter has sought to widen nurses' and midwives' understanding of the origins, application and potential benefits of MT as a form of treatment. The underlying objective has been to encourage nursing and midwifery professionals to incorporate forms of MT into their work practices. A number of strategies have been provided to assist nurses to incorporate simple aspects of MT in a knowledgeable and effective manner. The best way to put MT into action is to start to experiment and follow your instinct with one or two approaches or techniques. Once you start to get responses and assess the impact music can have, then seek to make MT part of your daily interaction with patients.

Make music part of your own daily lifestyle. Surround yourself with your favourite music. Allow it to be a source of 'soul food' and use it to nourish your mental, physical and spiritual being. If you personally connect to the therapeutic elements of music it will be much easier for you to extend this learning and apply it to patient care with enthusiasm and conviction.

ACKNOWLEDGMENTS

I am sincerely grateful to Joel Barolsky, Pauline McCabe and Tammy Rabinowicz for their contribution to this chapter and their ongoing support and encouragement.

REFERENCES

Albert NM (1996): Commentary on music therapy: a nursing intervention for the control of pain and anxiety in the ICU: a review of the research literature. *AACN Nursing Scan in Critical Care* 6(3):1-2.

Baily P (1973): *They can Make Music.* Oxford University Press.

Benenzon RO(1993): *Music Therapy Manual.* St Louis: MMB Music Inc.

Brewer JF (1998): Healing sounds. *Complementary Therapies in Nursing and Midwifery.* 4(1):7-12.

Brown CJ, Chen CAN, Dworkin SF (1989): Music in the control of human pain. *Music Therapy* 8:47-60.

Campbell D (1991): *Music and the Physician for Times to Come.* USA: Quest Books.
Clark ME, Lipe AW, Bilbrey M (1998): Use of music to decrease aggressive behaviors in people with dementia. *Journal of Gerontological Nursing* 24(7):10-17.

Curtis SL (1986): The effect of music on pain relief and relaxation of the terminally ill. *Journal of Music Therapy* 23(1):10-24.

Davis WB and Gfeller KE and Thaut MH (1992): *An Introduction to Music Therapy.*
Ellis DS, Brighthouse G .(1952): Effects of music on respiration and heart rate. *American Journal of Psycholog.* 65:39-47.

Ezzone S, Baker C, Rosselet R, Terepka E (1998): Music as an adjunct to antiemetic therapy. *Oncology Nursing Forum* 25(9):1551-1556.

Holmberg SK, Coon S (1999): Ambient sound levels in a state psychiatric hospital. *Archives of Psychiatric Nursing* 13(3):117-126.

Lai Y (1999): Effects of music listening on depressed women in Taiwan. *Issues in Mental Health Nursing* 20(3):229-246.

Lloyd-Green L (1990): The Role of the Music Therapist in Australia in the 1990s as a Member of the Allied Health Multi-Disciplinary Team in Palliative Care. Paper presented to the VIIth International Music Medicine Symposium, Melbourne, Victoria July 12-15:1998.

Megel ME, Houser CW, Gleaves LS (1998): Children's responses to immunizations: lullabies as a distraction. *Issues in Comprehensive Pediatric Nursing* 21(3):129-145.

Menuhuin Y(1972): *Theme and Variations.* Heinemann.

Nordoff-Robbins (2000): Home Page *http://www.nordoff-robbins.com.au/* Accessed January 28th 2000.

Peggie A (1981): Musical Adaptation. *The Times Educational Supplement* 12(6).

Podolsky E (1945): *Music For Your Health.* New York: Bernard Ackerman.

Spintge R. (1993): Music and surgery and pain therapy. Paper presented at the Joint North American Conference on Music Therapy. Toronto. Canada.

Standley JM (1998): The effect of music and multimodal stimulation on responses of premature infants in neonatal intensive care. *Pediatric Nursing* 2(6):532–540.

Stratton VN and Zalanowski AH (1984): The relationship between music, degree of linking and self reported relaxation. *Journal of Music Therapy* 21b, 184–192.
Tame D (1984): *The secret Power of Music.* Vermont, USA: Destiny Books.

Trauger-Querry B, Haghighi KR (1999): Balancing the focus: art and music therapy for pain control and symptom management in hospice care. *Hospice Journal: Physical, Psychosocial and Pastoral Care of the Dying* 14(1):25–38.

Updike PA (1998): Opening to the sacred: intentional use of music to engage the spiritual dimension. *Advanced Practice Nursing Quarterly* 4(1):64–69.

White JM (1999): Effects of relaxing music on cardiac autonomic balance and anxiety after acute myocardial infarction. *American Journal of Critical Care* 8(4):220–230.

Wiand NE (1997): Relaxation levels achieved by Lamaze-trained pregnant women listening to music and ocean sound tapes. *Journal of Perinatal Education* 6(4):1–8.

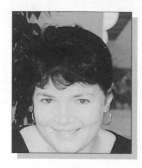

KIRSTEN JAMES
RN, Bachelor of Arts (Social Sciences), Graduate Diploma in
Adult Education and Training, Graduate Diploma in Healing
Therapies, Certificate of Tactile Therapies (Relaxation
Massage)

Freelance lecturer and consultant in private practice, and
registered nurse at Mount Alexander Hospital, Castlemaine,
Victoria

Kirsten was introduced to complementary therapies when working
in the UK some 10 years ago. Western medicine emphasises
medications and surgery as the cornerstones of health care. Kirsten
believes that complementary therapies offer a broader, more holistic
range of treatment options. She also believes they offer more scope
to individualise care, and the opportunity for people to acquire
means of empowering themselves and accepting responsibility for
their own health. In 1995 she established a consultancy to facilitate
the safe and professional introduction of complementary therapies
into a variety of health care settings.

Kirsten lectures in complementary therapies at RMIT and Victoria
Universities in Melbourne. She is currently undertaking a master's
degree at the latter university exploring why nurses choose
complementary therapies. Kirsten lives in country Victoria and
would like to thank 'Rennie the Wonderdog' for his support whilst
she was writing this chapter.

Chapter 14

Nursing and the role of animals

> ... *to be healthy, it is necessary to make contact with other kinds of living things ... If people are to come to terms with their own animal nature, they must feel the rest of the living world around them.*
>
> (Beck and Katcher, 1996:xiv).

INTRODUCTION

Humans and animals have evolved together over thousands of years to the extent, one could argue, that a relationship of co-dependency exists (Newby, 1999). Animals play an important part in many cultures throughout the world. They are used for protection, work, assisting people with disabilities, and companionship. Other examples of the ways in which animals are used by humans include:

- breeding animals for food production (either the animal itself or its by-products, e.g. milk, eggs)
- police work, such as drug detection, crowd control, search and rescue
- clothing and accessory/equipment manufacture (use of the wool, fur, skin or hide)
- skin care and cosmetics (lanolin, emu oil)
- scientific research
- teaching our children values such as care and responsibility, and educating them about sexual reproduction and death.

A more recent development has been to acknowledge animals as a therapeutic modality that can improve health outcomes in humans. A number of research studies provide clear evidence that human–animal interaction yields numerous benefits (Anderson et al., 1992; McHarg et al., 1995; Anderson, 1996; Heady, 1999; and Moody, 1999). This chapter explores the impact of animals on human health and discusses how nurses can facilitate pet therapy into health care.

HISTORY

As stated previously, the history of human and animal interaction is a long one, spanning many thousands of years. However, when refining the subject down to specific health interactions, we can begin with the 'father of medicine', Hippocrates (460–377 BC), who apparently wrote about the importance of 'natural exercise', which included horse riding.

It is not until 1792 that we find written reference to pet therapy by the Quakers in England. They founded the York Retreat as an alternative to the lunatic asylums of that time, and records indicate that animals were used at the retreat for therapeutic purposes. Patients could 'learn self control by having dependent upon them creatures weaker than themselves' (Beck and Katcher, 1996:132).

The Bethel Centre was an establishment that treated people with epilepsy in Bielefeld, Germany. Documents have revealed that, in the late nineteenth century, pets were used at the centre as an integral component of patient treatment. In 1944, patients at the Army Air Corps Convalescent Centre in Pawling, New York, were encouraged to interact with the animals on the centre's working farm, as part of an organised program.

However, it was American Boris Levinson PhD, who pioneered pet therapy and coined the term 'pet-oriented psychotherapy'. Dr. Levinson was the first professionally trained clinician to formally introduce companion animals and document the way in which they could be used as an adjunct in the practice of psychology. He advocated the use of animals in cases where affection and unconditional acceptance were indicated, and acknowledged that ' . . . pets satisfy vital emotional needs' (Levinson, 1969, in Perelle and Granville, 1999).

Levinson's compatriots Elizabeth and Samuel Corson, PhD, initiated 'pet-facilitated therapy' or PFT in the psychiatric hospital of Ohio State University in 1967 with considerable success (Padus, 1992). In the previous year, 1966, a blind gentleman, Erling Stordahl, established a rehabilitation centre in Norway for people with disabilities. Exercise and many other physical activities such as skiing were taught and encouraged through the use of horses and dogs (Beck and Katcher, 1996).

The first world congress on pet therapy was held in England in 1980 and since then, a number of organisations have emerged, including:

> North American Association of Pet Facilitated Therapists
> Delta Society, Animal-Assisted Therapy Services (USA)
> Pets as Therapy, UK (charitable organisation)

Visiting Pet Service (Australia)
Riding for the Disabled (worldwide)

There are a number of other, often voluntary, organisations and smaller community groups that offer guided and supervised interaction activities involving humans and animals.

DEFINITIONS AND SCIENTIFIC RESEARCH

The term 'pet-facilitated therapy', coined by Levinson some 40 years ago, has been superseded by the broader and more accurate 'animal-assisted therapy' (AAT). However, it should be noted that animal–human interaction can be considered therapeutic in both formal and informal ways. Simply observing animals, even watching documentaries, can be beneficial to the viewer, but actual interaction with animals appears to have more impact. Talking to an animal, holding or petting it, and taking it for a walk are commonly accepted ways that humans interact with animals. Humans probably underestimate the importance of the sometimes 'intimate' nature of the relationship. For example, taking a shower or sharing personal thoughts or feelings are activities that may occur only in the presence of particular friends or family members. To be able to behave naturally, with complete freedom, without fear of criticism or judgement, can mean that such simple interactions are examples of the therapeutic value of animals (Dillow, 1996; and Beck and Katcher, 1996).

> *Relating to animals means learning to communicate across the species barrier. When that communication is based on touch, trust, and gentleness, it can be truly life-enhancing, as it seems to call forth a very ancient link.*
>
> (Davis, 1999:125).

Academic interest in how animals influence human behaviour, lifestyle and health has grown in recent years, with the number of dissertations, research studies and journal articles notably increasing (Davis, 1999). Five universities in the USA alone have programs dedicated to the animal–human bond, and thousands of nurses, psychologists, social workers, educators, diversional and occupational therapists are involved in a range of modalities. The bonding process is what differentiates therapy from entertainment (Beck and Katcher, 1996).

An increasing number of studies are revealing support for a range of therapeutic claims associated with pet therapy that were previously based on anecdotal and empirical data. The benefits can be categorised as physical, psychological and educational.

215

Physical

Benefits include:

- improvement in mobility and fine and gross motor skills
- improvement in standing balance (Delta, 1999)
- lowering of blood pressure and serum triglyceride levels (Anderson et al., 1992; and Katcher et al., 1984 in Serpell, 1996)
- promotion of physical activity due to a pet's need for feeding and exercise (Padus, 1992; Beck and Katcher, 1996; and Davis, 1999)
- reduction of muscle tension and regulation of blood glucose levels through the promotion of relaxation (Pizzorino and Murray, 1994)
- reduction of pain through the comfort, warmth and texture of the animal's body and coat (Montagu, 1978; and Delta, 1999)
- improved recovery and survival rates following surgery and hospitalisation for conditions such as heart disease (Friedman and Thomas, 1995 in Anderson, 1996)
- reduced medication use in cardiovascular disease amongst pet owners (Heady and Anderson, 1995)
- over the course of a year, pet owners had fewer visits to general practitioners compared with people without pets (Bricklin, 1990, in McCormack, 1993; and Serpell, 1996).

Psychological

Benefits include:

- reduction in insomnia, stress and depression
- improved self-esteem, social contacts and ability to empathise (Serpell, 1996; and Davis, 1999)
- improved willingness to be involved in group activities
- reduction in the number of fights and suicide attempts in prisons (Davis, 1999)
- opportunity for comfort and nurturing
- more resilient to the effects of bereavement (Akiyama et al., 1987; and Bolin, 1987, in Serpell, 1996)
- improvement in communication and confidence
- improved sense of safety, security and independence (Beck and Katcher, 1996)
- valuable distraction and source of amusement which can promote play and lift the spirits (McCaul and Malott, 1984; and Beck and Katcher, 1996)
- feeling of acceptance—animals accept people without qualification and they do not care about appearance; they are non-judgemental and uncritical
- a bridge is created for patients who are withdrawn, uncooperative and uncommunicative (Delta Society, 1999)
- opportunity for non-threatening physical contact and tactile sensations that may have been difficult with humans, e.g. victims of abuse (Montagu, 1978; and Davis, 1999).

Educational

Benefits include:

- aiding long- and short-term memory
- increasing vocabulary
- understanding concepts such as responsibility and accountability (Delta, 1999)
- improving knowledge of concepts such as size and colour
- learning about sexuality, reproduction and birth
- helping to deal with the concept of death (James, in Snyder and Lindquist, 1998).

Some people also claim that animals can promote *spiritual* fulfilment. These people sometimes describe a sense of connection with nature and/or their God when observing or interacting with animals, particularly in a natural environment (Beck and Katcher, 1996; Delta Society, 1999; and Davis, 1999).

Scientific reasons for using animals as legitimate therapeutic health tools include psychoneuroimmunology and endorphins.

Psychoneuroimmunology

Sometimes called 'mindbody medicine' this science has helped to give credence to the connection between thoughts, attitudes and emotions and their direct impact or influence on the body at a cellular level. The comfort, companionship, security and love that an animal can provide to a human is therefore not to be overlooked as a very real means of providing health benefits in a truly holistic sense (Dillow, 1996; Beck and Katcher, 1996; and James, in Snyder and Lindquist, 1998).

Endorphins

'Mother nature's narcotics', endorphins, are stimulated when humans do something they enjoy, or when they exercise, laugh or cry. Therefore, if people enjoy undertaking any of the observational or interactional opportunities available with animals, endorphins will be stimulated. The reason this effect is important is that endorphins can impact on wellbeing in a number of ways, including reducing pain, stimulating the immune system and altering mood (Padus, 1992; and Hoptman and Hoptman, 1996).

RELAXATION

As mentioned previously, relaxation is recognised as having numerous benefits and can be readily stimulated with human–animal interaction or observation. More details about relaxation can be found in Chapter 11.

According to Benson and Stuart (1993) and Pizzorno and Murray (1994), relaxation outcomes include:

- reduction in blood pressure, heart rate and breath rate
- decreased inflammation, swelling and pain awareness
- less worry, more confidence and control
- improved quality of decision making and memory.

PRECAUTIONS

The important factor to keep in mind about the impact of animals on human health is that, as for any complementary therapy, a therapeutic effect is unlikely if the person has some negative memory association or is allergic to animals. Therefore, individual choice and awareness of past experiences with animals are key issues that the health care professional needs to consider when determining the appropriateness of pet therapy for a patient, resident or client.

As with a number of complementary therapies, there are some drawbacks to animal therapy, particularly pet ownership. The responsibility of owning a pet means there are costs associated with adequately feeding, housing and maintaining the animal (for example, vaccinations and grooming). A person's freedom can be limited, because someone has to take care of the pet in the owner's absence. Pets can be noisy, smelly, dirty, incontinent, sick, aggressive, destructive and sexually hyperactive, which can make them an embarrassment and nuisance to their owner. Bites and scratches are also inherent risks in owning an animal. Hundreds of thousands of injuries caused by animals and requiring medical treatment are documented annually in the UK and USA (Serpell, 1996:14–16).

However, in the context of animals being used by health professionals for therapeutic purposes, particular attention can be paid to the animal's personality and cleanliness to avoid potential problems. The specific issues to consider are detailed later in the chapter. It would appear that, if planning and preparation are undertaken, the beneficial outcomes far outweigh the potential risks.

Specific modalities involving animals, birds and fish are many and varied but can include the following:

- Riding for the Disabled is a voluntary group that provides horse riding lessons for children and adults with disabilities for recreation, sport, education and therapy (Stephens, 1999).

- Hippotherapy is a specialised medical therapy in which the client is placed in a number of positions and actively responds to the movement of the therapy horse. The therapist directs the horse's movement, analysing the client's response and adjusting treatment accordingly. It is used to improve balance, mobility and function (James, in Snyder and Lindquist, 1998).
- Rehabilitation of convicted criminals can occur, for example, through horse-breaking and/or caring for injured wildlife. Criminals have often experienced dysfunctional and sometimes violent relationships with humans, but can develop loving, constructive relationships with animals, which improves their communication skills (Davis, 1999).
- Zoos, reservations and sanctuaries are excellent places to visit.
- Bird watching can be done almost anywhere.
- Whale watching has become very popular.
- Swimming with dolphins is available in some places.
- Listening to (live or recorded) animal sounds, e.g. whales, dolphins, birds, frogs and even insects (crickets and cicadas) can be very therapeutic.
- Aquariums are known to be relaxing.
- Service animals, usually dogs, are individually trained to work or perform tasks for a person with one or more disabilities, e.g. vision or hearing impaired, epilepsy, mobility (Delta Society, 1999).
- Animal-assisted therapy (AAT) (see below).
- Animal-assisted activities (AAA) (see below).
- In 1995 statistics showed Australia to have the highest pet ownership rate per capita in the world—66% of all households owned a pet. Americans spend an estimated US$19 billion annually feeding, housing, caring and indulging their pets (Beck and Katcher, 1996).

Essentially, the concept of animal–human interaction as a therapy suggests that the animals are the force that enhances treatment and/or care, and it can be undertaken on an informal basis or on a formal basis. An example of the latter is seen with animal-assisted therapy (AAT).

The formal definition of AAT is:

> *AAT is a goal-directed intervention in which an animal that meets specific criteria is an integral part of the treatment process. AAT is directed and/or delivered by a health/human service professional with specialised expertise, and within the scope of practice of his/her profession, AAT is designed to promote improvement in human physical, social, emotional, and/or cognitive functioning ... AAT is provided in a variety of settings and may be group or individual in nature. This process is documented and evaluated.*
>
> (Delta Society, 1999).

AAT is a formal process and must contain the following three characteristics:
1. It is directed by health/human services professionals as a normal part of their practice.
2. It is goal directed.
3. It is documented.

Animal-assisted activities (AAA) were adapted from AAT and are not as formal. An example is the casual 'meet and greet' activities such as pet visitation that currently occurs in hospitals, hospices and aged care facilities. AAA also includes residential situations where an animal lives in a facility permanently. The same activities (e.g. petting, playing, feeding, walking) can be repeated with more than one person unlike an AAT program that is specifically tailored to suit an individual or medical condition.

The formal definition of AAA is:

> *AAA provides opportunities for motivational, educational, recreational, and/or therapeutic benefits to enhance quality of life. AAA are delivered in a variety of environments by specifically trained professionals, paraprofessionals, and/or volunteers, in association with animals that meet specific criteria.*
>
> (Delta Society, 1999).

AAA does not necessarily fulfil all three of the characteristics outlined for AAT.

NURSING AND ANIMALS

The literature indicates that the role of nurses and midwives in helping to facilitate human–animal interaction has been in existence in the USA for a lot longer than in Australasia. In the latter, it has largely occurred on an ad hoc basis until recent times. Often the involvement of nurses and midwives appears to have been by default, rather than something that is formally structured and organised. Many nurses, I suspect, are totally unaware of the existing and potential benefits that animals can have for their patients, residents and/or clients.

The presence of animals, in a residential and/or visiting capacity, appears to be on the increase in a number of settings where nurses and midwives work, including hospital wards (adult, paediatric, acute and extended care), hospices, nursing homes and hostels (low- and high-care facilities), rehabilitation centres, prisons and psychiatric settings. Nurses and midwives often initiate new care programs; at the very least they should be involved in an observational capacity because of the implications for direct patient care. Directors of nursing often become involved when issues such as infection control and/or the need for policy development arise. Policy development for pet therapy programs will be addressed in more detail in the next section of the chapter. Details about developing guidelines can be found in Chapter 3.

An increasing number of Australasian hospitals and aged care facilities have included animals in some way in their environment, to enhance patient or resident wellbeing. At Karoonda Hospital in country South Australia, 'Harold', the resident golden retriever, gives comfort to the elderly residents living in the aged care facility. Staff report that the dog intuitively gravitates towards ill or dying residents. At Mount Alexander Hospital in Castlemaine, Victoria, the two resident cats stroll around particular areas in the hospital, while a low key visiting dog program has been implemented for the aged-care residents living in the low- and high-care facilities.

The Alfred Hospital in Melbourne runs a successful visiting dog program in their palliative care unit. The dogs have their own photo identification badges. Dr. Wendy Moody introduced the first formal visiting program for in-patients at the Mater Children's Hospital in Brisbane. Formal policy guidelines were developed for Dr Moody's program and are reproduced with permission as Appendix 14.1 at the end of the chapter.

GUIDELINES FOR NURSING INTERVENTIONS

It is advisable to take into consideration the professional implications of introducing complementary therapies into health care settings. This should include any involvement of animals, whether it is an informal visitation program run on an ad hoc basis or a formal animal-assisted therapy program.

Legal and ethical issues are involved and the health and safety and individual rights of the patients and staff members must be considered in keeping with relevant nursing codes of conduct throughout the world. There are some risks associated with animal contact in general, but very few reports of any adverse effects occur in the literature (Beck and Katcher, 1996:131).

The following guidelines may be helpful to those who are considering initiating a pet program or for those who already have residential or visiting animals but have not yet drawn up formal documentation. The guidelines are not intended to be prescriptive, but are meant to raise some important considerations.

GUIDELINES FOR VISITING AND RESIDENTIAL ANIMAL PROGRAMS

- Consider the suitability of pet therapy programs in your particular workplace, for example, space, layout, carpet quality and the opportunity for privacy.
- Consult all key stakeholders or their representatives about the pros and cons of such a program, and anticipate any potential problems. Issues such as allergies to dog hair or cat fur, cultural objections, and negative memory associations should be flagged before the program is initiated.
- Consider the costs involved, including the purchase of the animal, vaccinations and veterinary care, regular health checks, food, toys, grooming and bedding equipment.
- Devise a policy that includes issues such as:
  - Responsibility for the animal (feeding, training, control, exercising and grooming needs).
  - Infection control issues (vaccination, vet-checks, prophylactic medications, cleaning and reporting of pet soiling, exclusion issues for certain patients e.g. immunocompromised and those with open wounds).
  - Insurance coverage for any unforeseen liabilities arising from accidents with the animals.
  - Qualifications and suitability of the animal handler who may be visiting the institution, e.g. cheerful personality, well-groomed with effective communication skills, able to follow health care facility policies and honour confidentiality.
  - Choice of the animal, for example, health status check, temperament assessment, grooming and cleanliness.
  - Documentation of animal–patient interactions and any outcomes—incident reporting and protocols for accidents such as dog bites, cat scratches, pet soiling.
  - The issue of feeding the animals—sometimes the health of the animal can be compromised from over-feeding or inappropriate feeding by well-intentioned residents or patients.
  - The name and contact details of a suitably qualified and experienced animal therapy consultant should the need arise (James, in Snyder and Lindquist, 1998:290; Moody, 1999; and Delta Society, 1999).

Protocols for visiting pets may include the following

- Keep dogs on leads at all times and in control of the handler or person taking responsibility.
- Some handlers encourage the use of food treats to help the animal get to know the client, but guidance about the suitability of treats may be required.
- The receptiveness of the client is important and can be assessed by observing client reactions and asking their opinions.

- Rather than persisting with clients who may be indifferent, allow the animal to spend 'quality time' with patients who respond positively (James, in Snyder and Lindquist, 1998:291).

CONCLUSION

Increasing research and empirical data clearly indicate that human–animal interactions can have a considerable therapeutic impact on the psychological, physical and spiritual wellbeing of humans. Therefore, animal assisted therapy is entitled to be considered a legitimate complementary therapy by nurses, midwives and other health professionals. However, considered planning and thought needs to be undertaken to successfully implement an animal program, either residential or visiting, with attention paid to individual choice and risk minimisation.

ACKNOWLEDGMENTS

The author is grateful for professional contributions to this chapter from Dr Wendy Moody, animal-assisted therapy consultant, Queensland, and input from Dr Malcolm Ramsay, veterinarian, Victoria.

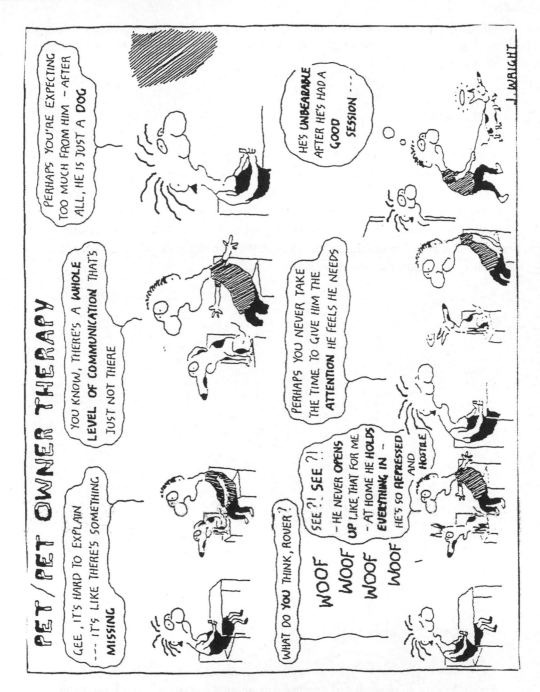

Figure 14.1: So, pet ownership can be stressful!

The cartoon is reproduced with the permission of the cartoonist, John Wright and the *Age* newspaper.

ENDNOTE

Things we can learn from a dog

- *Never pass up on an opportunity to go for a joy ride.*
- *Allow the experience of fresh air and wind in your face to be pure ecstasy.*
- *When loved ones come, always run to greet them.*
- *Let others know when they have invaded your territory.*
- *Take naps and stretch before rising.*
- *Run, romp and play daily.*
- *Eat with gusto and enthusiasm.*
- *Be loyal.*
- *Never pretend to be something you are not.*
- *If what you want is buried dig it up.*
- *When someone is having a bad day—be silent, sit close by and nuzzle them gently.*
- *Thrive on attention and let people touch you.*
- *Avoid biting when a simple growl will do.*
- *On hot days, drink lots and rest under a shady tree.*
- *When you are happy, dance around a lot and wag your whole body.*
- *No matter how often you are scolded, do not buy into the guilt thing— run right back and make friends.*
- *Bond with your pack.*
- *Delight in the simple joy of a long walk.*

Author unknown.

APPENDIX 14.1

ANIMAL-ASSISTED THERAPY WITHIN HOSPITALS
SUGGESTED INFECTION CONTROL—A SUMMARY

Reducing health risks in:
- the animal
- patients
- volunteers
- the location.

The animal

All dogs should be up-to-date with vaccinations and have a current veterinary certificate. Routine puppy vaccinations should be done at six, twelve and sixteen weeks. Dogs should be vaccinated for distemper, hepatitis, parvovirus, parainfluenza and bordatella, and should be revaccinated every year for the same diseases.

All dogs must be free of ecto- and endo-parasites such as monitor pathogens. Swabs should be taken every two months from the nasopharynx for streptococcus; the rectum for culture and sensitivity and ova, cysts and parasites. If necessary skin and hair scrapings can be taken.

All dogs must be on preventative medication for hookworm, toxicara (roundworm), tapeworm, heartworm and whipworm.

All dogs should be washed and vacuumed prior to each visit and kept in a clean area.

Any soiling should be cleaned up immediately by a volunteer who carries a plastic bag. The incident should be reported to the nurses and soiled areas disinfected as for human faeces.

Volunteer

A pre-program health check and vaccination update should be attended to. Written agreement regarding responsible behaviour is required and encompasses:
1. reporting ill health in self or pet and exclusion from hospital until recovered
2. general hygiene e.g. handwashing after each patient
3. control of the pet within the hospital
4. cleaning up and reporting pet soiling
5. wearing a covering garment.

Patient

The medical team should give permission for pet visits and permission should be recorded, along with the consent of the patient/parent/guardian/child on the admission forms.

Animals may be excluded from visiting patients with immunodeficiency states, oncology patients, those with burns or open wounds, patients in ICU and those with allergies to dogs.

Location

Visiting areas should be defined, for example, are pets allowed in designated areas only, wards only, outpatients departments, carpeted or uncarpeted areas, or all departments of the hospital? The areas from which pets are excluded should be defined. It should be clear whether dogs are allowed on beds, and if so, if an undercover is required.

© Therapeutic Solutions PTY LTD—Dr Wendy Moody MBBS PhD 1998

redsoil@one.net.au

REFERENCES

Akiyama H, Holtzman JM, Britz WE (1987): Pet ownership and health status during bereavement. *Omega: Journal of Death & Dying* 17:187-93.

Anderson WP (1996): The Benefits of Pet Ownership. *The Medical Journal of Australia* 164:441-442.

Anderson WP, Reid CM, Jennings GL (1992): Pet ownership and risk factors for cardiovascular disease. *The Medical Journal of Australia* 157:298-301.

Beck A, Katcher A (1996): *Between Pets and People—the Importance of Animal Companionship* (revised edn). Indiana: Purdue University Press.

Benson H, Stuart EM (1993): *The Wellness Book.* New York: Fireside.

Davis S (1999): Our pets, ourselves. Spiritual lessons from the animal world. *Yoga Journal* January–February 53-57:123-126.

Dillow KA (1996): Pets and the elderly. *New Horizons* March–April:5-6.

Heady B, Anderson WP (1995): Health cost savings: the impact of pets on Australian health budgets. South Yarra, Victoria: Pet Information & Advisory Service.

Hoptman N, Hoptman C (1996): *HELP—Health Enhancement Lifestyle Program*. Alexandria, NSW: Millennium Books.

McCaul KD, Malott J (1984): Distraction and coping with pain. *Psychological Bulletin* 95:516-33.

McCormack GL (1993): *Pain Management—Mindbody Techniques for Treating Chronic Pain Syndromes*. Tuscon, Arizona: Therapy Skillbuilders.

McHarg M, Baldock C, Heady B and Robinson A (1995): National People and Pets Survey. Sydney, NSW: Urban Animal Management Coalition.

Moody W (1999): Hospital patients cheered up by dog visits. *Australian Doctor* 9 July.

Montague A (1978): *Touching* (2nd edn). New York: Harper and Row.

Newby J (1999): *The Animal Attraction*. Sydney, NSW: ABC Books.

Padus E (1992): *The Complete Guide to Your Emotions and Your Health*. Emmaus, PA: Rodale.

Perelle IB, Granville DA (1999): Assessment of the Effectiveness of a Pet Facilitated Therapy Program in a Nursing Home Setting. New York: Dept Psychology, Mercy College.

Pizzorno J, Murray M (1994): *Encyclopedia of Natural Medicine*. London: Optima.

Serpell J (1996): *In the Company of Animals: A Study of Human–Animal Relationships* (Canto edition). Cambridge: Cambridge University Press.

Snyder M, Lindquist R (1998): *Complementary/Alternative Therapies in Nursing* (3rd edn). New York: Springer Publishing Co.

Stephens J (1999): Ponies as Therapy. *Pets & Vets Australia* 1 10:44-47.

The Delta Society (1999): About Animal-Assisted Activities and Animal-Assisted Therapy. *Rrs.envirolink_org/psyeta/sa/sa1/perelle.html*. Accessed March 24th 2000.

Section Three

Complementary therapies in action: stories from the workplace

The information in Sections One and Two is drawn together in this final part of the book. Four clinicians describe their experiences of integrating complementary therapies into their workplaces from inception as a vision of enhanced practice to successful integration some years later. The journeys were not always easy. Nevertheless, in each case the benefits for patients, nurses, midwives, other practitioners, carers, and the healing environment itself have demonstrated the validity of using complementary therapies. Aromatherapy is obviously the most popular therapy with nurses at present. It is instructive to discover how each of the clinicians in Section Three has incorporated the therapy into practice and policy. The stories also provide insight into the use of complementary therapies in acute coronary care, midwifery, palliative care and aged care settings. In each case the authors were the primary initiators of complementary therapies in their work environments, extending nursing and midwifery practice and providing fine examples of nursing leadership. The chapters are inspiring and scholarly as well as pragmatic and offer a range of strategies, rationales, guidelines and practical advice for others wishing to follow the same road.

Chapter 15, **Complementary therapies in a high-tech health care environment: a pleasing and powerful partnership,** demonstrates very successfully that complementary therapies are not just for low-technology nursing environments. Marcia George is Nursing Unit Manager of the Coronary Care Unit of a major Melbourne teaching hospital. Her story describes the staff's journey from a situation of demoralisation to the provision of advanced holistic care that includes complementary therapies. The story makes inspiring reading. Coronary care is an environment that demands the highest standards in research and care. The use of complementary therapies has demonstrably improved the quality of care and the healing environment. The response from patients, relatives and staff has been 'extraordinarily positive', and the model of coronary care developed by Marcia and her staff has received international interest.

Chapter 16, **Complementary therapies in aged care**, offers nurses an alternative for managing the challenging behaviours of clients with dementia. Suzanne Thomson is the Director of Nursing and Aged Care Services at The Cedars Nursing Home in Casino, northern NSW. Staff in this unit found that many problem behaviours in residents could not adequately be addressed by conventional medical and nursing means. The nurses confronted their own frustration and demoralisation in a pro-active way by investigating the uses of aromatherapy in dementia care. The result has been a highly successful model of care that is now being exported to other aged care facilities. Suzanne provides a comprehensive coverage of the CT policy and documentation used at The Cedars. The case report of the use of aromatherapy in the care of one wandering and agitated resident makes very interesting reading.

Chapter 17 is titled **Complementary therapies in a palliative care setting: the clinical experience.** In this chapter Rose Osborne, Clinical Nurse at Daw House Hospice in Adelaide, provides a comprehensive insight into the incorporation of various complementary therapies into the hospice, and the development of complementary care as a model of nursing practice. Rose was instrumental in setting up a freestanding complementary care centre at Daw House where inpatients and outpatients are able to access the benefits of complementary therapies. The establishment of this centre and the resulting increased scope of nursing practice are described. One interesting treatment used at Daw House, aromatic hot towel compress and abdominal massage, blends three different therapies and is described in detail. The chapter ends with the findings of a research project to evaluate complementary care at Daw House.

Chapter 18, the final chapter of the book, is **Complementary therapies in midwifery practice.** Susie Nanayakkara has previously written a book on baby massage and brings her considerable midwifery experience to bear on the integration of complementary therapies into the Birth Unit at Auburn Hospital in Sydney, NSW. The chapter describes the background to the inclusion of aromatherapy in midwifery, and gives practical advice about useful essential oils, their effects, and precautions to be taken. The Birth Unit has now had nine years' experience using aromatherapy and the benefits of this CT for patients, staff, and the unit generally are described. These benefits include decreased use of narcotics by labouring women.

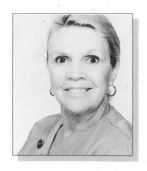

MARCIA GEORGE
RN, RM, Certificates in Intensive Care and Coronary Care
Nursing, Bachelor Applied Science (Nursing), Graduate
Diploma Human Relationships (Education), current study,
Master of Nursing–Converted to PhD Candidature

Marcia is currently the Nurse Unit Manager of the coronary
care unit at the Austin and Repatriation Medical Centre

Prior to her current role, Marcia held the position of charge nurse of
the intensive care and coronary care units at the Preston and
Northcote Community Hospital in Victoria between 1982 and 1991.
Her nursing experience also includes aged care, gynaecology and
maternity nursing, obstetrics and paediatrics and over two decades
of critical care nursing. Marcia has always believed that hospital
environments, in particular, high-tech health care environments, are
often viewed as austere and frightening by the general community.
She also believes that with a little imagination, and a relatively small
budget, a lot can be done to enhance and transform these
environments into health care areas that are more comfortable and
conducive to both the physical and psychological healing needs of
patients and their families. Marcia is married with two adult children
and two grandsons. Her interests include music, literature, bush
walking and golf.

Complementary therapies in a high-tech health care environment: a pleasing and powerful partnership

Create a dream and give it everything you have, you could be surprised just how much you are capable of achieving.

Sara Henderson (1995:4).

BACKGROUND INFORMATION

In order to fully appreciate why the transformation of a high-tech health care environment was considered in the first place, one needs to have an understanding of the complexity of the environment as well as the needs and clinical details of the patients being cared for in this environment. The following pages give an overview of cardiovascular disease and some aspects of its management in a coronary care unit that has been programmed for healing and promoting health.

CARDIOVASCULAR DISEASE

Cardiovascular disease (CVD), is largely preventable, yet it continues to be the leading cause of premature death and illness in Australia. One Australian dies every ten minutes as a result of CVD (Commonwealth of Australia National Goals, Targets and Strategies for Better Health Outcomes, 1994:xi).

Cardiovascular disease includes coronary artery disease, stroke, heart failure and peripheral vascular disease caused by damage to the blood supply to the heart, brain and legs. These conditions share common major risk factors, which include behavioural risk factors such as tobacco smoking, physical inactivity, poor nutrition, and high consumption of alcohol; and behavioural risk factors such as high blood pressure, overweight and obesity, elevated blood lipids and diabetes mellitus. Coronary heart disease is the most common CVD and remains the major cause of death in people under 70 years of age (Commonwealth of Australia National Goals, Targets and Strategies for Better Health Outcomes, 1994:xi).

THE IMPORTANCE OF EFFECTIVE CARDIAC REHABILITATION PROGRAMS

In the mid 1980's, Scandinavian medical researchers Hedback (1989) and Perk (1989) collaborated in a longitudinal study conducted over 10 years that measured the health outcomes of two groups of patients with acute myocardial infarction. Both groups of patients came from similar sociodemographic backgrounds, and were admitted to two separate but comparable hospitals. The first hospital, the control group, gave patients routine acute care and cardiac rehabilitation and secondary prevention. The second hospital, the experimental group, gave patients routine acute care supplemented by cardiac rehabilitation and secondary prevention. The results from this study demonstrated significant differences in health outcomes between the two groups. Patients who received routine acute care together with cardiac rehabilitation and secondary prevention programs:
- lived longer
- had fewer complications
- had fewer readmissions to hospital
- required less medication
- returned to work earlier
- had fewer psychosocial problems
- had better control of their blood pressure
- had better control of their cholesterol and serum lipids
than the patients who received routine acute care and no cardiac rehabilitation or secondary prevention program (Hedback, 1989; and Perk, 1989:47). In other words, secondary prevention programs can save lives and improve the quality of life and longevity of patients with cardiac illness.

The results of similar studies demonstrate the importance of providing cardiac patients with effective secondary prevention and rehabilitation programs. Up until this time, cardiac rehabilitation and secondary prevention programs received limited acknowledgment in mainstream health care. However, world health authorities such as the World Health Organisation (1993) and the National Heart Foundation of Australia

(1998) now advocate that all patients admitted to hospital with cardiac disease be offered cardiac rehabilitation and secondary prevention programs. The National Heart Foundation of Australia recently published minimum standards for cardiac rehabilitation programs.

Cardiac rehabilitation consists of three phases. Phase 1 takes place in the acute care setting and continues until the patient is discharged from hospital. Phase 2 occurs in the outpatient setting and requires the patient and family members to attend once or twice a week for a period of four to six weeks. Phase 3 involves long-term maintenance.

With reduced length of stay in hospital and early discharge, some health professionals believe that Phase 1 cardiac rehabilitation programs are ineffective and a waste of time. This point of view is based on the premise that patients are unable to retain the information offered in Phase 1 programs. However, for the nurses who work in coronary/cardiac care environments, and who are responsible for providing patients with Phase 1 programs, the beginning phase of cardiac rehabilitation represents a unique and powerful platform for health counselling.

Many cardiac/coronary care nurses believe that effective Phase 1 programs are the genesis of effective cardiac rehabilitation. To health professionals who advocate the benefits of Phase 1 programs, patients (and their families) are perhaps never more motivated than in the acute phase of their disease. It would be true to say that cardiac patients are often facing their own mortality for the first time in their lives. As a result, many of these patients are motivated to reflect on their lifestyles and risk factors and to make the very best of their second chance at life, health, and wellbeing.

The importance of Phase 1 programs is highlighted even further, when the numbers of eligible patients attending Phase 2 programs are considered. It has been estimated that fewer than half the patients who are eligible for a Phase 2 program actually attend. Of those who do attend, a substantial number do not complete the program (Commonwealth of Australia National Goals, Targets and Strategies for Better Health Outcomes, 1994:89).

Hence, if cardiac patients are not provided with Phase 1 programs, and fail to either attend, or complete two programs, there will be an increasing population of patients, who receive none or minimal cardiac rehabilitation. These sub-optimal attendance rates should be a concern to all health professionals working in cardiac care environments. The nursing group featured in this chapter considered it to be professionally and ethically unacceptable for patients not to be provided with individualised Phase 1 programs.

PHASE 1 PROGRAMS COMPROMISED BY HOSPITAL ENVIRONMENTS

The health benefits associated with effective cardiac rehabilitation have already been discussed. Yet, in practice, health professionals find that patients can be so overwhelmed by the seriousness of their illness and the complexity of their care in high-tech environments that they are unable to relate to, or retain, many of the vital health messages offered to them during their hospital stay. Perhaps this issue, together with markedly reduced time in hospital, may significantly compromise patients' long-term health and wellbeing.

PRIMARY PREVENTION

The admission of patients to coronary and cardiac care environments is generally a time of great concern and anxiety for their families and friends. Yet, with appropriate support and counselling, this stressful time can become a time of reflection. Common cardiac risk factors can be identified, along with ways in which the risks can be reduced. In addition, primary prevention offers the building blocks for lifestyle change. It can generate and harness the motivational energy required for lifestyle change to take place. Family members can be reassured, encouraged and given a sense of hope. In short, primary prevention has a vital role in preventing premature death and premature illness in the Australian community.

HIGH-TECH HEALTH CARE ENVIRONMENTS

Cardiac patients and their relatives can experience high levels of concern and anxiety during the early stages of their hospital admission (George, 1995:31). These concerns can be further exacerbated by the sights, sounds and sensations that accompany the plethora of complex medical technology that is now an integral part of the routine care and management of cardiac patients.

Technology in health care has been described by Bates and Linder-Pelz (1987:115) as being:

> *Essentially a tool outside the human body, which is used to perform a desired task. Medical technologies include drugs; anaesthesia; surgical procedures and instruments; devices implanted into the body; machinery to do tests, and the scientific knowledge which enables all these tools to be put to use.*

Medical technology is essential for saving lives and preventing many of the complications associated with cardiac disease. While medical technology is routine and commonplace for the health professionals who work in coronary care environments, for many patients and their relatives, high-tech health care environments appear alien, austere, depersonalising and frightening. Patients and families can be so overwhelmed by the complexity of the environment that they are unable to retain, or relate to, the vital health messages offered to them in primary and secondary prevention programs. As a result, long-term health outcomes may be seriously compromised.

Ironically, it seems the health care environments that were created to save lives and aid recovery, can actually affect the prognosis and impede optimal recovery. This viewpoint is supported by Guzetta (1989:609) who described the admission of a patient to the coronary care unit (CCU) with the presumptive diagnosis of acute myocardial infarction as a 'psychophysiologically stressful experience capable of adversely affecting the patient's prognosis and recovery'. The words of Curtin (1984:7) give further support to this argument: 'The more technological the environment—and the more technological the intervention—the greater the need for human contact, for human responses to fundamentally human needs.'

It was the levels of stress and anxiety experienced by cardiac patients and their families in a high-tech CCU, combined with nursing goals for improving the effectiveness of the cardiac rehabilitation program, that served as the catalyst for a group of critical care nurses to completely transform not only their CCU environment, but also, almost every aspect of their practice.

A CLIMATE OF CHANGE IN HEALTH CARE

In 1991 major changes occurred in the Victorian health care system. The Heidelberg Repatriation Hospital in Victoria was preparing for a change that would take it from being a Commonwealth funded hospital to a state funded hospital.

A short time later, it was decided that the Heidelberg Repatriation Hospital and its near neighbour, the Austin Hospital would be amalgamated into one major Victorian public hospital. Plans were announced for all health care services on both campuses to be consolidated. It was a time of massive restructuring and economic reform. These reforms heralded the closing of some departments, as well as early retirement plans, redundancy packages and many other changes to staffing and health services. This climate of change was challenging, and at times, extremely difficult for many health professionals. Morale seemed at times to reach a record low.

A CAREER MOVE IN A CLIMATE OF CHANGE

In late October 1991, and in a climate of massive health care change, the author embarked on a career move. Her decision was made despite many enjoyable and fulfilling years as charge nurse of a busy combined intensive care, coronary care and high dependency unit. The time now seemed right for pursuing a long held interest in coronary and cardiac nursing.

The author was appointed to the position of charge nurse of the Repatriation Hospital's CCU, and looked forward to a new challenge and the opportunity to develop her cardiac knowledge and skills. At the time, there was no way of knowing that an extraordinary journey of holistic discovery was about to begin, or that the journey would be shared with and exceptional team of critical care nurses.

The Heidelberg Repatriation Hospital's CCU had been without a permanent charge nurse for some period of time. The Unit was well overdue for some refurbishment. Additionally, there were many professional and practice issues in need of evaluation. Although a number of the CCU nurses had worked together for a considerable period of time, there was a general perception that team commitment and morale was fragmented and in need of improvement.

THE JOURNEY BEGINS

At first there was a substantial 'getting to know you' period. Focus group meetings, together with general group meetings, allowed practice and professional issues to be highlighted and openly and honestly discussed and debated. Initially, the concerns of the nurses dominated the meetings. For example, they raised concerns about:
• the future viability of the nursing team as they knew it
• the future viability of health services at the Repatriation Campus
• the future of colleagues in other departments
• the impact economic reform was having throughout the public health system
• the plummeting morale among health professionals and more specifically throughout nursing generally.

Following these discussions the nurses (from now on also referred to as the group), decided to adopt a pro-active approach to dealing with the massive changes they were confronting. This pro-active stance provided the group with a much needed positive focus. The group began an immediate review of all policies, protocols and nursing practices, which were either updated, or completely changed. A sense of renewed energy and commitment was evolving. At times, the energy and determination was almost palpable.

The season of change in health care had provided the group with a unique opportunity to explore new and innovative approaches to patient care. In this sense, economic reform paved the way for the group to reflect on their practice and then confidently begin an enlightening journey. The hallmarks of the shared journey will now be discussed.

IDENTIFYING HOLISTIC HEALTH CARE AS A COMMON VALUE AND BELIEF

Focus group discussions enabled common professional values and beliefs to be established. When analysed, these values and beliefs appeared to centre on the principle that nursing was based on a holistic philosophy and nursing practice should reflect a holistic model of care. However, articulating and defining exactly what was meant by a holistic model of care proved to be a difficult task.

The group began by searching the literature for an appropriate definition of holistic care. It was important for this definition to reflect the realities and complexities of the group's practice. Blatner (1981) discusses at length the issues surrounding holistic health and holistic health care. She highlights the difficulties associated with defining the relevant terminology.

The Nurses Reference Library defines holistic health care as:

> *A system of comprehensive or total patient care that considers the physical, emotional, social, economic, and spiritual needs of the person; the response to illness; and the impact of the illness on the person's ability to meet self-care needs*
> (Nurses Reference Library, 1985:457).

This definition eventually provided the framework for the nurses to develop their own definition of holistic health care, which will be discussed later in the chapter.

THE IMPORTANCE OF ENVIRONMENT

As stated earlier, the group was well aware of how high-tech environments can impact on patient care and patient outcomes. It soon became evident that a true holistic model of care would require significant environmental changes. The group was unanimous about the need to soften the technological and highly clinical ambience in the unit. The climate of change presented an opportune time for the group to explore the concept of providing a more 'healing' environment, in which state-of-the-art technology and the expertise and knowledge of medical and nursing specialists came together in a way that was conducive to the reflective and restorative needs of patients and their families; a health care environment that would be perceived as tranquil and comfortable, non-threatening and calming, with the essential clinical and technological aspects of care being softened and enhanced by elements from the patient's natural world. The colours, textures, sounds and smells should be in keeping with their every day lives.

This viewpoint is not a new concept. In fact, almost a century and a half ago, Florence Nightingale, in her best known work, *Notes on Nursing,* wrote 'Little as we know about the way in which we are affected by form, colour, and light, we do know this: They have an actual physical effect' (Nightingale, 1859:5). More recently, Brummelaar (1999) suggests that hospital environments need to be designed to accommodate the emotional needs of patients. She also argues that an important part of healing relates to how safe and comfortable patients feel. Likewise, Kaiser (1995:22) suggests wholeness is about curing and healing 'Whilst curing is about wholeness of body, healing is about wholeness of being.'

The literature supported the group's belief, that the environment has a profound effect on people's outcomes. Environmental transformation now became fundamental to their goals for developing a holistic model of care and healing ambience in the unit.

THE ART AND SCIENCE OF NURSING

Once the need for substantial environmental change had been identified, the group began examining ways of implementing a holistic approach to care in their unit. Although the group agreed that holistic care or 'whole person care' was integral to practice, there was ambivalence about exactly how a holistic model of care could be effectively applied in practice. Questions were raised: How does holistic care differ from routine care? How can patients and others in the health care team identify holistic care? How can holistic care be visible? These questions emphasised the group's need for further clarification about the role of nursing in a contemporary and rapidly changing health care arena.

Many nurse authors, including Henderson (1966), have described nursing as both an art and a science. In high-tech health care environments the science associated with nursing and patient care can be glaringly obvious. Unfortunately, however, the art of nursing is not always so readily apparent or acknowledgeable.

To many nurses who have worked, or continue to work in high-tech health care environments, it seems as though the priorities of care are sometimes focused on the science and technology, rather than on the human being who is dependent on the technology. This viewpoint is supported by the comments of a retiring medical director of a major intensive care unit in Melbourne who described his dismay at what he termed as 'hi-tech, low touch medicine in critical care environments' (Suzuki (1990:57). Taylor (1999:31) stated 'Technology has enormous benefits. They are undeniable—that's why we're hooked on it.'

The group's next undertaking was to ensure that both the art and the science of nursing were being represented in a balanced approach to practice. They identified three primary levels of patient care, requiring three primary levels of nursing. These separate levels of care became known as scientific care, humanistic care and environmental care, safety and integrity (George, 1991). The three separate levels of care were then defined and promoted as a contemporary representation of both the art and the science of nursing.

SCIENTIFIC CARE

Scientific care is the level of care requiring the expertise of nursing and medical specialists and state-of-the-art medical technology. It considers the anatomical, physiological, pathological, biochemical and technological health care needs of patients. Scientific care includes the most basic health care technology such as catheters, feeding tubes, oxygen cannula, pharmaceutical products, and lifting devices, as well as the most sophisticated and complex medical technologies.

Scientific care represents a major part of contemporary health care, and is essential for saving lives, curing illness, aiding recovery, improving quality of life, and for reducing some of the complications arising from health problems, both cardiac related and other. Scientific care and best practice standards in health care require health care professionals to have their scientific skills, knowledge and competency levels regularly updated and evaluated (George, 1993; 1994; 1998; 1999).

HUMANISTIC CARE

Humanistic care describes the level of care required to meet the individual and holistic needs of patients, and includes their psychological, emotional, social, economic, vocational, cultural and spiritual needs (George, 1993; 1994; 1998; 1999). Humanistic care requires health care professionals to practise with a well developed, culturally sensitive, mature, caring and empathic commitment to individualised patient care (George, 1998;1999).

The importance of meeting the humanistic needs of patients is supported by Hare (1986) who argues that the successful rehabilitation of cardiac patients is more likely to be related to psychological (humanistic) factors rather than physical (scientific) factors. This viewpoint is given further support by Seldon (1986:395) who argues that:

> *Australian reports and many overseas studies on cardiac rehabilitation make the point that the extent of invalidism after cardiac illness relates more to psychological factors than to the severity of the heart disease.*

In essence, it is now a well recognised fact that failure to meet the psychological and emotional (humanistic) needs of patients can result in cardiac patients suffering with many more problems of the 'mind' than of the 'heart' following cardiac illness.

THE THREE LEVELS OF CARE CENTRAL TO A HOLISTIC MODEL OF CARE

Further discussion and reviewing of the literature and practice convinced the group that an effective holistic model of care was a dynamic continuum of care that systematically assessed and endeavoured to address the humanistic, scientific and environmental health care needs of individual patients. These three separate levels of care were incorporated into a conceptual framework that is depicted in Figure 15.1.

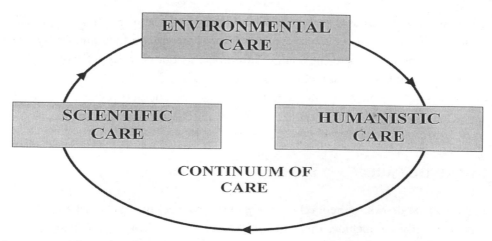

Figure 15.1: Three levels of care central to a holistic model of care (George, 1992)

Once the conceptual framework had been identified, the group's next goal was to develop a definition of holistic nursing that was relevant to the complex and clinical needs of the group as well as the individual health care needs of the patients being cared for by the group. The definition that eventually evolved was:

> *Holistic nursing in a contemporary health care environment, endeavours to provide for the individual, humanistic, scientific, and environmental health care needs of patients; by promoting, and providing a balanced, systematic, and comprehensive approach to patient care, nursing practice, and health education.*
>
> (George, 1993; 1994; 1998).

The group believed that the key words contained in this definition encompassed the primary principles of both their practice and their holistic philosophy of care. They were satisfied that their definition was relevant. and it was incorporated into to the mission statement of the CCU, which was printed, enlarged, framed and then hung in a prominent place in the unit. It reads as follows:

> *We endeavour to provide, promote and further develop a cohesive nursing team, committed to the pursuit of clinical excellence and the highest standards of individualised holistic patient care.*
>
> (George, 1994).

The group believed that best practice standards of care, and optimal patient health outcomes, were dependent on a balance of care that considered and endeavoured to meet the humanistic, scientific and environmental needs of patients. This balance in care is required 24 hours a day, seven days a week. The nursing profession is the only profession that offers this level of care in this constant time frame. Hence, it was again highlighted to the group that the role of nursing is fundamental to achieving balanced care.

TRANSFORMING A HIGH-TECH HEALTH CARE ENVIRONMENT

The environmental needs of patients and the impact of health care environments on patient outcomes has been discussed. The CCU environment had been a source of concern for the nursing staff for some time, and the time was right for them to move to the next stage of their holistic journey. Despite the closure of wards and downsizing of departments throughout the public health system, there was a feeling of excitement and challenge within the group. The transformation of the CCU was about to unfold. There was no blueprint to work from and the changes that evolved were based solely on intuition.

MORALE AND FINANCIAL SUPPORT

Support, financial and moral, was sought from management and various charity groups working for the hospital. Many letters outlining the group's vision for the future of the unit were written and forwarded to appropriate departments within the hospital. The response was encouraging. It seemed that most people approached were able to appreciate the vision and the rationale for transforming the unit. Approval and financial support from the hospital enabled the transformation to commence.

THE CRITICAL CARE ENVIRONMENT PRIOR TO TRANSFORMATION

Like most critical care environments there was a plethora of high-tech equipment, with complex visual and sound effects. The walls and drapes in each patient cubicle were a beige colour. Cupboard doors and joinery throughout the unit were either grey or dark blue in colour. The main central area was carpeted in a dark brown, rather worn carpet. Although all patient areas had external windows there were no clocks or pictures on the walls. Stark fluorescent lighting operated 24 hours a day. Essentially, the unit's decor was very clinical and technical.

FOLLOWING TRANSFORMATION

The gradual transformation of the unit included the following:
- Soft pastel colours were introduced throughout the unit, including the softest of pinks and greens.
- The bright fluorescent lighting was replaced with subdued, indirect lighting (emergency and clinical examination lighting was retained).
- Artwork that features an Australian native flora theme was hung throughout the patient care areas.
- Numerous pot plants with artificial foliage were placed throughout the unit.
- A two-hour daily patient rest period was introduced.
- The brown carpet was replaced with new pastel coloured carpet.
- New hydraulic patient beds with luxury mattresses were purchased and the stark blue quilts were replaced with pastel coloured textured quilts.

The transformation was well under way and the unit looked beautiful. The soft pastel decor, together with indirect lighting, environmental prints and pot plants, had made an extraordinary difference. Patients, staff and visitors were all offering favourable comments.

At that point, the unit's transformation was entirely visual. Yet, as previously discussed, the group were well aware that high-tech health care environments can impact negatively on all of the human senses—sight, sound, touch, taste and smell. The group realised that in order to provide a true 'healing' environment, there needed to be some means by which all of the human senses could be reached and connected with in a positive way. At this stage the role of complementary therapies was first considered.

THE INTRODUCTION OF COMPLEMENTARY THERAPIES

Complementary therapies and complementary care, according to the position statement of the Royal College of Nursing, Australia (RCNA), (1997), are 'understood to be an approach to health care which recognises the principles of holism and complementarity as they apply to health, nursing, healing and therapeutic interventions'. In retrospect, the RCNA position statement served to reaffirm the group's foresight in introducing complementary therapies to practice so many years ago (early in 1992–1993). The nurses began to take great pride in the knowledge that they were trailblazers in an exciting approach to patient care. Perhaps it is worthwhile restating that the transformation took place in the early 1990s, when the typical high-tech environment appeared to be dominated by a highly clinical, scientific, and technological paradigm. The concept of complementary therapies was very controversial and virtually unheard of at that time.

Very early in the unit's transformation other health professionals began to ask certain questions such as, 'Where is the scientific evidence that complementary therapies are effective?', and 'Where are the double-blind, randomised, controlled studies proving the efficacy of complementary therapies?' Although such questions were relevant, they were almost impossible to answer because of the paucity of complementary therapies research. Despite the scepticism, there was general acceptance that complementary therapies were enhancing patients' perceptions of care, and doing no harm, so the use of complementary therapies in the unit continued.

The growing popularity and wide acceptance of some complementary therapies in the unit has enabled other complementary therapies to be introduced. The unit now promotes and provides: music, relaxation, massage and aromatherapy. These complementary therapies are specifically used to target the human senses of sight, hearing, touch and smell.

MUSIC

It was with the human senses and the human spirit in mind that music became the first complementary therapy introduced to the unit. With the support of management a compact disc (CD) player and a selection of CDs were purchased. In addition, individual patient 'walkman' tape cassettes were purchased. This equipment enabled appropriate music to be incorporated into the routine care and management of patients. Music has continued to have a central focus in the unit because: 'Within the boundaries of the health care institution, the sounds of illness become the only song that is heard unless the environment is programmed for healing' (Kerfoot, 1993:1).

When appropriate, and with the availability of 'walkman' devices, the nursing staff introduced patients to relaxation music and tapes. Some of the staff were qualified to teach relaxation techniques. It is interesting to note that many patients continued to use relaxation tapes and include relaxation techniques in their day-to-day health maintenance plan following discharge from hospital. In this sense, complementary therapies helped empower patients and encouraged them to take an active interest in maintaining their own health and wellbeing.

AROMATHERAPY

Although in the early 1990s most of the nurses in the unit had probably heard or read a little about aromatherapy, none had actually experienced or been involved in aromatherapy in any way. One day, the unit's newly appointed ward clerk, also a qualified aromatherapist, approached the nursing staff to discuss the potential use of aromatherapy. At first, aromatherapy seemed far too controversial but following careful consideration, much discussion, and an extensive literature search, aromatherapy was introduced to the unit. It was immediately an outstanding hit with patients, visitors, and the multi-disciplinary health care team. Within a few days staff were requesting more information and the wider use of aromatherapy in the unit.

Aromatherapy now has a major role in the unit's healing environment and in patient care. Guidelines for the use of aromatherapy and massage are included later in the chapter.

MASSAGE

> We often talk about the way we talk, and we frequently try to see the way we see, but for some reason we have rarely touched on the way we touch.
>
> (Morris, 1971:3).

Massage was introduced to the unit next. Some nurses already had formal massage qualifications, others were either enrolled or considering enrolling in massage courses. Hence, when and where appropriate, massage was increasingly being used as an adjunct to routine patient care. Furthermore, from time to time, staff can be seen giving each other head and neck, upper back or hand massage. This practice continues to grow and is particularly prevalent during times of increased levels of stress in the unit.

RESEARCH

The role of complementary therapies and the environmental changes that took place in our unit have been validated in a collaborative research project. The research evaluated nurses' perceptions of the efficacy of complementary therapies in a high-tech coronary care unit. The results have not yet been published, but they clearly demonstrate that nurse clinicians believe complementary therapies add a valuable dimension to their practice, promote a holistic philosophy of care, improve standards in patient care, contribute to improved patient outcomes, and provide nurses with a sense of empowerment and professional worth (Scott and George, 1998).

ADVERSE REACTIONS

Despite the wide acceptance of complementary therapies a few staff members experienced some minor reactions, such as headache, nausea and watering eyes, to some of the essential oils. These reactions were generally the result of an inappropriate choice of essential oils, or using too much essential oil. They serve to highlight the need for and importance of guidelines for the use of complementary therapies. Guidelines were developed and implemented and have enabled the safe use of complementary therapies to be continued and enjoyed by patients, visitors and staff for the past seven years or more.

GUIDELINES FOR THE USE OF COMPLEMENTARY THERAPIES

Aromatherapy
Essential oils that can cause adverse reactions are:
* peppermint *(Mentha piperita)* (nausea)
* cedarwood *(Cedrus atlantica)* (dizziness and bronchospasm)
* lavender *(Lavandula officinalis)*, ylang ylang *(Cananga odorata)* and geranium *(Pelargonium graveolens)* (headache when used in excess).

From the experience gained in the unit, there are a number of recommendations.

- Lavender and orange *(Citrus aurantium)* are the unit's basic oils of choice.
- Less is best for maximum benefit; only a few drops of essential oil are necessary. It is important to realise that any more than a few drops could result in an adverse reaction.
- Responsibility for aromatherapy, including the integrity of the various electrically powered aromatherapy vaporisers used in the unit, is very important. Following discussion, a consensus agreement resulted in the decision that the RN in charge of each shift would be responsible for the choice, blend and safe vapourising of the essential oils being used. The nurse in charge can delegate this responsibility to another staff member where and when applicable.
- The use and choice of essential oils to be used for the forthcoming shift is decided following discussion after nursing handover. This practice enables staff to be aware of which oils are being used and the specific needs and sensitivities of patients and staff can be safely accommodated.
- It is recommended that essential oil vaporisers be checked following the routine policy checking of dangerous drugs at the beginning of each shift. This helps ensure consistency with the quality use of aromatherapy and continuity with important checking procedures.
- A decision not to vapourise essential oils during the shift is acceptable provided the vapourisers are empty and turned off at the power point.
- The specific essential oils being vapourised in the unit are indicated on an *'Essential oils in use'* notice board. Hence, staff and visitors to the unit are informed about exactly which essential oils are being vapourised.
- Qualified and experienced practitioners can use a range of essential oils according to the needs and individual choices of patients and staff members.

Patients are informed of the unit's use of aromatherapy and other complementary therapies as soon as possible after admission. Consent to use aromatherapy in the patient's immediate environment is generally sought while taking the patient's health history. The consent, or refusal to consent, is documented in a specific section of the history. So far, after seven years of using complementary therapies, only one patient has requested that aromatherapy not be used in his environment.

These guidelines, together with a sensible and cautious team approach to aromatherapy have enabled the financial costs associated with the use of essential oils to be absorbed into the general running costs of the unit. For more detailed information about aromatherapy see Chapter 9.

Massage therapies

Massage is not a new concept in nursing. It has been at the centre of nursing's traditional 'back wash' for decades However, other forms of massage are now used in patient care, for example, therapeutic, relaxation and sports massage. These forms of massage have been widely promoted in the general community and throughout many health environments. The benefits of massage are well recognised. Yet, massage, like most other therapies, also has some side effects in some individuals.

It is therefore important for nursing practitioners who include, or are planning to include massage therapies in their nursing practice, to be well aware of not only the benefits, but also some of the potentially negative responses that can be induced with some forms of massage. The side effects of massage can be divided into two distinct categories:

- physical side effects, such as soft tissue injuries when inappropriate massage techniques and therapies are performed when the patient has an underlying injury and/or disease processes
- psychological side effects, such as those that can occur when massage therapy includes imagery or visualisation techniques—these side effects are most likely to occur with emotionally vulnerable individuals.

Until the nursing profession can substantiate and support the use of complementary therapies with reputable research results, the following practice guidelines are recommended:

1. A comprehensive health history should be obtained prior to using any complementary therapy.
2. Fully assess the patient prior to using any complementary therapy and at least once each shift according to the clinical condition.
3. Obtain informed consent.
4. The use of imagery or visualisation in massage should be undertaken only by health professionals with appropriate qualifications, competence and expertise.
5. Nurses who intend to incorporate massage into their practice should consider undertaking a formal massage course or structured in-service program.
6. Non-fragrant, basic oil should be available for massage. It is recommended that lavender be the only essential oil added to the basic massage oil unless the practitioner is a qualified aromatherapist and has the patient's consent to use other essential oils (George, 1998, 1999).

These simple complementary therapy guidelines enabled complementary therapies to be implemented and widely accepted as contributing to quality standards of patient care in a very busy, mechanistic, critical care environment. So far there have been no adverse reactions or negative responses from the patients being cared for in this environment.

> *When you are in a healing environment, you know it; no analysis is required.*
> *You somehow feel welcome, balanced, and at one with yourself and the world.*
> *You are both relaxed and stimulated, reassured, and invited to expand. You feel*
> *at home.*

(Venolia, 1995:5).

CONCLUSION

Although the coronary care unit featured in this chapter has closed, most of the original members of the nursing group are working together in a newly developed unit on the Austin Campus of the Austin and Repatriation Medical Centre. The new unit has all the features of the original unit, such as specifically chosen colour schemes, music, plants, environmental prints, massage and aromatherapy.

It also has added features such as a compact disc music system that can be tailored to individual patients' needs and a closed circuit audio-visual system for relaxation and health counselling sessions. In addition, artwork which features Australian native flora has been incorporated into feature wall plaques and decorative wall borders. Bed linen has been specifically chosen to coordinate with the unit's colour scheme.

Once again, the feedback from nurses, patients and the multi-disciplinary team has been extraordinarily positive. The unit's environment and use of complementary therapies continues to attract interest from health professionals both nationally and internationally. The principles underpinning the group's holistic model of care have been incorporated into a patient assessment tool as well as all policies, protocols, nursing handover information and nursing documentation. A stringent cleaning and infection control program accompanies this holistic model of care.

In essence, a holistic model of care, together with a common sense approach to the use of complementary therapies, and the promotion of a healing environment, has enabled this nursing group to remain united and focused, with a strong sense of worth and common purpose during a particularly difficult time in health care history. Perhaps another point of interest is that, despite the enormous amount of change this nursing team has experienced, the attrition rate among these nurses remains consistently low.

These nurses have shown that when state-of-the-art medical technology is supported with the expertise of health care specialists, a holistic model of care, and an improved health care environment, optimal patient health outcomes can be achieved. Indeed, the experiences of these nurses has clearly shown that high-tech health care and complementary therapies can be effectively combined to provide a powerful and pleasing partnership in health care.

The shared experiences of these nurses has been likened to a remarkable holistic journey. During this journey, the patients the nurses cared for, together with the family members they supported and the health professionals they worked beside, have expressed their appreciation of the holistic model of care and importantly, the difference it made to their lives. The experience also made a difference to the way in which these patients, their family members, and the multi-disciplinary team now view the role of professional nursing and its contribution to the health and wellbeing of the community as a whole.

Nursing has realities to face: new concepts [in] health care, its own history, its own nostalgia and that of associated professions, its own education. Only if these are faced can nursing develop in all its dimensions and release the creative possibilities of all its practitioners.

(Nahm, 1971:13).

ACKNOWLEDGMENTS

This chapter is dedicated to a special group of nurses who kept alive what seemed to some to be almost an impossible dream. Together, and with a shared and collective sense of determination, these nurses systematically transformed a highly clinical and high-tech health care environment.

Together, we dared to be different. We challenged long held, rigid and conventional norms. We overcame the barriers, the self-doubts and the scepticism. Our reward has been so sweet. Our vision is now reality. We have succeeded in proving to ourselves, our patients, and our colleagues, the power of holistic nursing, and importantly, just how professional nursing makes a difference in health care. Others now follow.

REFERENCES

Curtin L (1984): Nursing: High-touch in a high-tech world. *Nursing Management* 15:7:7–8.

Bates E and Linder-Pelz, S (1987): *Health Care Issues.* NSW. Australia: Allen & Unwin Pty Ltd, p. 115.

Blatner B (1981): *Holistic Nursing.* Englewood Cliffs, NJ: Prentice-Hall, Inc.

Brummelaar H (1999): The People of Design. *Hospital and Healthcare.* May:8–9. Surrey Hills New South Wales, Australia: Yaffa Publishing Group Pty Ltd.

Commonwealth of Australia (1994): *National Goals, Targets and Strategies for Better Health Outcomes into the Next Century.* Canberra: Commonwealth Department of Human Services and Health, p. xi.

George M (1991): Prototype of Humanistic and Scientific Care. Paper presented to the First National Conference on Nursing Diagnosis, held in Queensland, December.

George M (1993): Defining holistic nursing in a contemporary health care environment and developing a nursing mission statement. Heidelberg Repatriation Hospital. Heidelberg, Victoria: Coronary Care Unit.

George M (1994): . Nursing Diagnosis—A Theoretical Concept Undermining Clinical Credence. Paper presented to the Second National Nursing Diagnosis Conference held in Western Australia, December.

George M (1995): Nursing framework for cardiac rehabilitation. *Collegian* (2)2:29–33.

George M (1998): Guidelines for the use of complementary therapies in a high-tech coronary care unit Developed for the coronary care unit, Repatriation Campus, Austin and Repatriation Medical Centre, Heidelberg, Victoria (unpublished).

George M (1999): Updating of guidelines for the use of complementary therapies in a high-tech coronary care unit, Austin Campus, Austin and Repatriation Medical Centre, Heidelberg, Victoria.

Guzzetta C (1989): Effects of relaxation and music therapy on patients in a coronary care unit, with presumptive acute myocardial infarction. *Heart and Lung* 18(6):609–616.

Hare D (1986): Cardiac rehabilitation. Notes on cardiovascular diseases. National Heart Foundation (Victorian Division), West Melbourne. February (22):1:1.

Hedback B (1989): Cardiac rehabilitation after myocardial infarction and coronary artery surgery. Linkoping University Medical Dissertations No296, Sweden.

Henderson S (1995): *From Strength to Strength.* Pan Macmillan Publishers. Australia, p. 4.

Henderson V (1966) *The Nature of Nursing.* New York: Macmillan Co

Kaiser L (1995):The centre for innovation. St Lukes Episcopal Hospital. Houston,Texas. *Innovator* Spring/Summer edition, p. 22.

Kerfoot K (1993): St Lukes Episcopal Hospital. Division of Nursing. Houston,Texas. *Innovator* Spring edition, p. 1.

Morris D (1971). In Autton N (ed.) *Touch and Exploration.* London: Darton, Longman and Todd Ltd, p. 3.

Nahm H (1971): Nursing Dimensions and Realities. In: Lewin E (ed.). *Changing Patterns of Nursing Practice—New Needs, New Roles.* New York:The American Journal of Nursing Company.

National Heart Foundation of Australia (1998): *Directory of Cardiac Rehabilitation.* Canberra: National heart Foundation.

Nightingale F (1859 reprinted in 1946): *Notes on Nursing.* Philadelphia, PA: Edward Stern & Co. Inc.

Nurses' Reference Library (1985): Definitions. Nursing 85 Books. Springhouse Corporation. Springhouse, PA, p. 457.

Perk J (1989): Cardiac Rehabilitation. Linkoping University Medical Dissertations No 295, Sweden.

Taylor T (1999):An intensive career. Saturday Interview with Dr Bernard Clarke. *Herald Sun.* Saturday, 23 October, p. 31.

Royal College of Nursing,Australia (1997): Guidelines for the Use of Complementary Therapies in Nursing Practice. RCNA: Canberra ACT.

Scott S and George M (1998): Evaluating nurses' perceptions of complementary therapies in a high-tech coronary care unit. Research project undertaken in the coronary care unit and the Repatriation Campus of the Austin and Repatriation Medical Centre (in press).

Seldon W (1986): Simplifying cardiac rehabilitation (editorial). *Medical Journal of Australia* April 14; 144(8):395.

Suzuki D (1990): *Inventing the Future.* Sydney:Allen & Unwin, p. 57.

Venolia C (1988): *Creating Healing Environments.* Berkley, CA: Celestial Arts.

World Health Organisation (1993): Report of Expert Committee on Rehabilitation after Cardiovascular Diseases.WHO Technical Report Series No 831.WHO, Geneva.

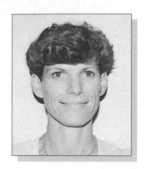

SUZANNE THOMSON
RN, Bachelor of Health Management (UNE)

Director of Nursing and Aged Care Services, The Cedars Nursing Home, A Project of the Frank Whiddon Masonic Homes of New South Wales

Suzanne completed general nurse training at Tamworth Base Hospital, New South Wales, in 1982. Since then she has worked in the acute and aged care sectors in public and private facilities in Queensland and New South Wales, gaining a diverse range of clinical and management experience. Since entering the nursing home industry in 1996, Suzanne has become passionate about issues that impact on aged care, and is committed to elevating the profile of nursing homes in general. She is equally committed to promoting professional practice in nursing homes to overturn the negative stigma associated with aged care nursing. She is resolute in her belief that staff empowerment is fundamental to its achievement. At present, Suzanne is a master's candidate (honours) at the University of New England, researching teamwork and organisational structures in residential care facilities.

Complementary therapies in aged care

INTRODUCTION

Health is a dominant value in Western society, permeating every aspect of people's lives. It induces individuals to demand medical treatment when illness occurs and passively accept the diagnosis and prognosis of scientific investigation, the so-called biomedical model of care. Taken to its extreme, the biomedical model of care assumes that the health care needs of older people are homogenous and require uniform management (Howe, 1985). The biomedical model does not fully recognise the intricacies and complexities of the ageing process. Numerous strategies have been designed by state and Federal governments in the last decade to overcome this problem (Sax, 1990). Nonetheless, it is apparent that approaches to the assessment, investigation and treatment of older people differ from other age groups. Many illnesses confronting older people in residential care facilities are regarded as sequential processes of ageing and reinforce the notion that age is equated with disability and illness (Davis and George, 1993).

Because older people are perceived to have lived beyond the roles of income earner, parent and spouse, they are consciously and unconsciously labelled by society as unproductive (Brown, 1994). Subsequently, health care professionals often incorrectly assume that older people are admitted to residential care facilities because medical intervention has failed, and further treatment is neither available nor effective. Anecdotal evidence suggests that health care professionals view aged care facilities as the 'end of the line'. Ultimately, nursing homes under the biomedical paradigm become the designated place of death.

A heterogenous approach to care is required to successfully address the issues that emanate from caring for older people in residential care facilities (Sax, 1990). Holistic or social approaches to care, focusing on the total individual, encompass a comprehensive range of variables that have the potential to positively impact on the health status of an older person. As society discovers that scientific medicine does not provide curative treatment for certain conditions, and fails to meet the psychological and spiritual needs of individuals, complementary therapies will augment their health care choices (Bates and Linder-Pelz, 1992).

This chapter has three fundamental objectives. It aims to demystify aged care nursing and aromatherapy, and simultaneously describe a recognised collaborative and integrated approach to care, involving complementary therapies, nursing care and medical science in an aged care facility. Finally, it aims to make a significant contribution towards raising the profile of aged care nursing.

WHY AROMATHERAPY?

The fundamental objectives of the Commonwealth Government's 1997 policy reform in the residential aged care sector were to improve standards of care; protect the civil rights of older people; streamline funding arrangements; and emphasise accessible, appropriate and affordable care (Department of Health and Family Services, 1997). In real terms, this resulted in funding constraints, excessive documentation requirements, expensive and complex accreditation processes and incongruent state and Federal legislation. These factors, combined with the inherent complexities associated with ageing, ensure that nurses in aged care facilities are faced with enormous challenges that medical science and government agencies do not address. Managing behaviour problems is a challenge.

These issues, in association with the continual quest of nursing professionals to have aged care nursing recognised as a unique speciality, and the perpetual pursuit of best practice, have provided The Cedars staff with the impetus to forge new ground in aromatherapy. Lavender oil vapourising was introduced at The Cedars under the guise of aromatherapy some time ago, primarily to eliminate unpleasant odours emanating from residents' rooms and dirty utility rooms. As a consequence, staff associated aromatherapy with captivating the olfactory senses. However, during the last couple of years, aromatherapy has transformed the holistic care processes at The Cedars.

The word 'holistic' is often interpreted as an idealistic mode of care that is shrouded in mysticism and embedded in theory. This social or holistic paradigm defines the whole individual as the central focus of care, rather than placing the focus on illness, disease or disability. Further, as Davis (1994) succinctly states, 'To restrict their care to the treatment of physical symptoms alone is inadequate and reductionist in nature'. The Cedars has developed a definitive holistic approach to care, where the total social identity of the residents is carefully considered when planning care. This heterogenous approach to care has allowed staff to embrace aromatherapy as an effective care modality.

Aromatherapy is used in The Cedars for:
- sleep disturbance
- aimless wandering
- anxiety
- relaxation
- skin allergies
- massage.

The case study presented at the end of the chapter indicates that further investigation into the application of aromatherapy is warranted.

The methods of application include inhalation from a vapouriser or from application to clothing and bed linen, chest rubs and massage. Currently, 53% of residents at The Cedars are having some form of aromatherapy.

The non-invasive nature of aromatherapy had a decided impact on the perceptions of health professionals, residents and representatives at The Cedars about its potential to be used as an effective treatment option. Scientific medicine, by its very nature, is invasive and many older people find this overwhelming, especially when they perceive their psychosocial needs are being disregarded. As older people discover that scientific medicine does not provide curative treatment for specific conditions, and fails to meet their psychological and spiritual needs, they willingly try aromatherapy as an alternative, or as an integral part of their treatment. Certainly, it has been the experience at The Cedars that residents and their representatives are more than willing to participate in aromatherapy treatments.

The impetus for the increased use of aromatherapy was largely a result of a series of factors that included:
- a supportive organisational management that encouraged staff empowerment, motivation and innovation
- an intense personal interest in aromatherapy by a core group of staff
- challenging resident behaviours that were unsuccessfully managed by medical and traditional nursing care.

Challenging behaviours are a primary focus of care delivery in residential care facilities. In an ideal world (utopia), residents with challenging behaviours could be managed without medical intervention. Appropriately designed accommodation, improved staff-to-resident ratios, and human and material resources that allow consistent program management are examples of ideal solutions. Realistically, many facilities are precluded from considering some, or all, of these options for a variety of reasons. Funding is the main constraint and The Cedars is no exception.

Behaviour management strategies are accorded a high priority at The Cedars. Actually, it has been the experience at The Cedars that not all behaviours can be managed successfully using behaviour management programs. Three important underlying issues associated with the complexity of managing challenging behaviours are:

- Each resident who comes to live in the nursing home comes with unique, indelible personality traits.
- Residents with challenging behaviours associated with dementia exhibit unique symptoms that are dependent on the area of the brain affected.
- Finally, as Sherman (1991) states, ' . . . the same illness may have different symptoms in different people.'

Residents exhibit a variety of repetitious behaviours that require complex, integrated management strategies, which are time consuming, strenuous and stressful for staff. These factors result in behaviour management revolving around the configurations of nursing home rituals and treatments, which depersonalise individuals (resulting in ' . . . blunted emotions') and reduce behaviour management ' . . . to a set of organisational exigencies' (Davis and George, 1993).

As a result of the difficulties in managing behaviour problems the nursing staff began to show signs of stress, such as frustration, hopelessness and agitation. These feelings gave way to nonchalance, as they recognised their attempts to solve the seemingly unsolvable were consuming valuable time and energy. The nursing staff sensed that the system had overwhelmed them. Ultimately, the potential was there to destroy staff morale, nursing practice and clinical confidence.

THE AROMATHERAPY COMMITTEE

A core group of staff became pro-active, using aromatherapy skills acquired over a period of time. The core group consisted of four committed nurses who established an aromatherapy committee specifically convened to investigate aromatherapy as an alternative care option and provide resources for personal care attendants and or professional staff.

Initially, the group was confronted with some resistance, scepticism and non-compliance. Resistance to change, for personal, social or professional reasons, was recognised as a crucial threat to the success of the aromatherapy program. Resistance to change is an inherent human phenomenon. It may become protracted, particularly when the security of accustomed practices is directly threatened and replaced with uncertainty, scepticism and non-compliance (Auer et al., 1993). It is often easier to resist change than to acquire new skills, develop alternative strategies or actively participate in or contribute to a clinical program where the outcomes are entirely unknown. It was therefore necessary to instigate staff education programs and to explain in detail the purpose and perceived benefits of the aromatherapy program. Aromatherapy education is now incorporated into The Cedars in-service program to build a knowledge base in aromatherapy practice and minimise the risks to residents and staff.

Members of the aromatherapy committee used non-confrontation consultation as a method of overcoming resistance to change. In particular, where the resistance was emanating from senior staff, their assistance to help formulate care plans was sought. This strategy proved very effective in breaking down barriers. It is interesting to note that the committee now provides informal advice about the therapeutic benefits of aromatherapy to 60% of staff and 25% of residents' relatives.

A major strength of the aromatherapy program is the possibility that staff, resident, representative and medical officer participation will improve compliance and therefore reduce complications and anxiety associated with illness. Ultimately, this may result in improved customer satisfaction and health status (Ewles and Simnett, 1992). In addition, the program has the potential to encourage working partnerships between health professionals that will generate closer alliances where each professional is valued for their skill and contribution. Effectively, this will also result in improved resident outcomes. Professionals involved in the program have the opportunity to increase their job satisfaction and career opportunities, which sets the foundation for increased productivity.

The specific responsibilities of the aromatherapy committee include:
• educating staff, residents and their representatives
• liaising with other local care facilities in the area regarding policies, procedures and aromatherapy practice
• assessing, planning and reviewing resident therapy
• producing monthly newsletters

- participating actively in regional meetings and forums on aromatherapy
- developing and reviewing policies and procedures
- accepting referrals
- investigating treatment options
- ensuring consent is obtained
- consulting with medical officers regarding treatment options
- maintaining competencies and staff education
- researching products
- developing quality management activities
- ensuring appropriate material and safety data information is available about all products.

THE CEDARS EDUCATION AND PROFESSIONAL DEVELOPMENT PHILOSOPHY

Professional development is accorded a high priority at The Cedars. Staff are provided with the opportunity to attend formal and informal education programs, internally and externally. This same commitment was extended to the aromatherapy program and the committee, and staff in general were actively encouraged to show initiative and creativity and to seek career guidance and advancement.

The objectives of the Cedars professional development program are to:
- promote flexibility, creativity and innovation in education and professional development
- nurture an environment that is conducive to staff education
- promote the acquisition of skills that allow staff to adapt to change and implement clinical models of best practice
- encourage professional competence
- evaluate education programs on a continuum
- introduce educational opportunities that will enhance clinical skills
- actively promote formal and informal continuing education
- identify relevant career paths and provide assistance to staff to help them achieve their career goals.

AROMATHERAPY POLICY AND PROCEDURE

The foundations of the aromatherapy policies and procedures at The Cedars are based on the position statements on complementary therapies of the Nurses Registration

Board of New South Wales and the New South Wales Nurses Association. Because aromatherapy as a recognised treatment modality is in its infancy in Australia, there were very few existing policies and procedures that the committee could use as the basis for The Cedars policies. Consequently, policies and procedures were being formulated and are evaluated on a continuum against recommendations made by the Nurses Registration Board, the New South Wales Nurses Association and other organisations actively involved in providing complementary therapies.

In addition, the aromatherapy policy statement and primary objective, as noted below, directly reflects The Cedars mission statement, its vision, values and objectives, which are known to all staff. Therefore, staff are able to readily relate to the fundamental purpose of the program.

AROMATHERAPY PROGRAM POLICY STATEMENT AND OBJECTIVE

The Cedars has adopted aromatherapy as a recognised complementary therapy and it is our policy to introduce essential oils, where required and appropriate, to enhance the quality of life of our residents.

Current policies and procedures cover the following issues:
- education
- professional standards
- quality management
- referrals
- assessments
- therapy intervention and therapy selection
- consent
- documentation
- aromatherapy practice
- storage and management of essential oils
- committee structure and terms of reference.

DOCUMENTATION AND CARE PLANNING (IN ORDER OF PROCEDURE)

- The *Aromatherapy Procedure Manual* outlines documentation and procedures at The Cedars.
- The resident history sheet must be completed within two weeks of admission.

Aspects of the resident's history are completed by the family with assistance given where required.

- An aromatherapy committee member should complete the aromatherapy care plan in consultation with the resident or their representative.
- The care plan must be endorsed by a second aromatherapy committee member.
- The resident's medical officer should be consulted about the proposed treatment and their approval obtained prior to the commencement of the therapy.
- Consent forms are completed by the resident and family/representative.
- A separate care plan is required for each condition treated.
- An essential oil allergy test should be completed 24 hours prior to use. Skin reactions and non-reactions must be documented in the progress notes. The test site is the inner wrist.
- Consider any aggression incident reports when implementing the resident's aromatherapy care plan.
- Assess unsettled dementia residents and record the results on a data sheet two weeks prior to the commencement of aromatherapy treatments.
- Data are to be collected for a further two weeks after the aromatherapy treatments commence, to gauge the effectiveness of the therapy. The program is then evaluated.
- Aromatherapy, other than for challenging behaviours, can be implemented after skin allergy testing and obtaining the consent of the medical officer and the resident/representative, and after the relevant documentation is completed.

It is important to note that the franchise nature of residential care facilities has resulted in a consumer driven industry that has become ' ... more litigious and complaint oriented' (New South Wales Nurses Association, 1999). Consequently, it is critical that documentation processes are definitive, conform with contemporary legal requirements and directly reflect organisational policy and procedures. Health care records can be put before a court as evidence or be examined by a court in any type of court proceeding (New South Wales Nurses Association, 1999).

In addition, records are a primary communication tool that define the objectives of care, the effects and outcomes of treatment and ultimately ensure continuity of care (Rorden and Taft, 1990). The aromatherapy request form (see Figure 16.1) is utilised to ensure that aromatherapy is not inappropriately initiated, altered or ceased. Recognising and conforming to documentation standards demonstrates quality care and provides a baseline from which the committee can formulate treatment options. Once the request form is completed, the committee builds a data base about the resident, which functions as a decision making tool, to help ensure continuity of care. Figure 16.2 illustrates the information compiled for each resident.

Next meeting:

Name	Date	B/P	Allergy	Epilepsy	Skin Irritant	Therapy Required For	Date Approved Signature

Figure 16.1: Aromatherapy request form. Requests are subject to approval by the Aromatherapy Committee

AROMATHERAPY HISTORY ASSESSMENT SHEET

Date: ____/____/____

Name: _____

Address: _____

Date of birth: ____/____/____   Male/Female: _____

Doctor: _____

Marital Status: _____

Previous medical history

	Yes	No
Blood pressure		
Urinary problems		
Present condition		
Accidents and/or operations		
Respiratory ailments		

Other assessments—considerations and precautions:

_____

_____

General health

Exercise/Leisure _____   Relaxation _____

Sight   _____   Hearing   _____

Hair   _____   Oedema   _____

Diet—detail e.g. diabetic: _____

Current medications:_____

Allergies:_____

Skin conditions:_____

Home stress

                                               Yes   No

Sleep pattern   _____   _____

Nervous condition   _____   _____

Phobia   _____   _____

Favourite colour: _____

Favourite aroma: _____

Signature of staff member requesting: _____

Signature of aromatherapy committee member:_____

Signature of registered nurse: _____

Figure 16.2: Aromatherapy assessment and history sheet

The assessment sheet is used to decide the most appropriate essential oil/s to be used and the method of application. The aromatherapy resident care plan is then formulated (see Figure16. 3). Planning the care of older people in high care facilities, who frequently have chronic diseases, becomes an important responsibility for nurses, and is frequently charged with emotion. The manner in which nurses effect their professional roles, within legal and ethical frameworks, is pivotal in ensuring optimal functioning of older people, regardless of the surroundings in which that care is administered (Johnstone, 1995). Therefore, a complete appraisal of the physiological and psychosocial needs of each resident is a central element in achieving that goal. The appraisal is primarily accomplished by the continuity of care process, in which adequate, timely, individualised care planning is effected. A plan of care that is explicitly individualised for each resident is developed, implemented and evaluated on a regular basis according to changes in resident care needs.

Attach patient label here.	**THE CEDARS NURSING HOME CARE PLAN** Aromatherapy		
Trial begin date: ____/____/____ Trial end date: ____/____/____	Resident specific		
	Allergy	Yes	No
	Skin irritant	Yes	No
	Blood pressure (high)	Yes	No
	Epilepsy	Yes	No
	Aggression incident report	Yes	No
	Skin test attended	Yes	No
Nursing/therapist diagnosis			
Outcome			
Interventions			
Evaluation Signed _____ Date _____	Alteration required New care plan formulated Yes No Yes No		
	Discussed with resident/ representative and health care team Yes No		

Figure 16.3: The Cedars nursing home care plan

CONSENT

It is important to note, although outside the scope of this chapter, ethical considerations and legal requirements were crucial considerations in The Cedars aromatherapy program. Nurses have a joint responsibility, with other health professionals, to provide residents and their representatives with relevant information, empowering them to make informed choices about the care they receive (Hartigan, 1987). This allows individuals the freedom and capacity to achieve and maintain optimal health outcomes. The issue of consent is therefore of paramount importance, both legally and ethically. As a criterion for quality care, residents and/or their representatives must be given information about their treatment programs, the objectives of the treatment and how it will be evaluated prior to commencing therapy. As the New South Wales Nurses Association (1999) states, 'People have a choice about whether or not they undergo a proposed operation, procedure or treatment and have a legal right to refuse to do so.' More detail about the legal and ethical issues relating to complementary therapies can be found in Chapter 5.

The following points are from The Cedars *Aromatherapy Procedure Manual*:
1. All residents and representatives will be provided with the relevant information required to make an informed decision about their treatment.
2. Residents at The Cedars, or their representatives, must complete the relevant consent form. (See Figure 16.4.).
3. The designated committee member, who is a registered nurse, will discuss the proposed treatment with the resident's medical officer and obtain their consent to instigate treatment.
4. All relevant documentation must be maintained in the clinical files.
5. With the addition of any essential oil or method of application, the consent of the resident or representative and the medical officer is to be obtained.

It has been noted that all medical officers caring for residents having aromatherapy treatments are very responsive, and some actively promote aromatherapy as a complementary therapy, or a treatment option. This attitudinal shift is possibly a result of the increasing frustration encountered by medical officers in addressing the complexities associated with ageing. In addition, The Cedars aromatherapy committee is working closely with the North Coast Aromatherapy Group to formulate a standardised consent form specifically for aromatherapy. Conventional medical consent forms do not adequately address complementary treatments or procedures authorised by medical officers and performed by nursing staff.

CONSENT FOR ROUTINE NURSING CARE

(A project of the Frank Whiddon Masonic Homes of NSW)
ACN: 082 395 091

Part A

RN_____ and I_____
      (Name of registered nurse)   (Name of resident/representative)

have discussed the nursing care needs of
_____
Name of resident

Please list nursing care—Part C:

The RN has also told me that:
• Additional procedures other than those explained to me and not noted in Part C may be required from time to time.
• It is often impracticable for nursing staff to contact me immediately to obtain consent each time a change in nursing care occurs.
• I acknowledge that I will be notified and consulted as soon as practicable regarding any change in standard routine nursing care.

_____   ___/___/___
      (Signature of resident/representative)

(Name of resident)

I, _____, RN, have informed the above as detailed.

_____
      (Signature of registered nurse)

Part B
I request and consent to standard/routine nursing care as described above for

_____
      (Name of resident)

except that I don't agree to having _____
           (Name of procedure)

If any additional standard routine procedures not explained to me or listed in Part C are necessary, I consent to these also.

_____   ___/___/___
      (Signature of resident representative)

(Name of resident)

_____
Signature of registered nurse

Part C

List of standard/routine nursing care

Routine nursing care involves, but is not limited to the following:
* application of continence appliances such as pads and uridomes
* application of standard skin emollients that are purchased over the counter at pharmacies/department stores
* application of alternative skin emollients that are made from herbal or other preparations
* instigation of aromatherapy treatments
* application of basic simple dressings such as Opsite to prevent friction or applied for protection
* eye care such as eye cleansing with normal saline
* changing fluid preparations from caffeinated preparations to decaffeinated preparations where the need has been indicated
* administration of nurse-initiated medication
* application of walk-belts and walking aids
* application of sheep skin to buttocks and feet
* utilisation of lifters and other manual handling equipment
* collection of urine/faecal/sputum samples
* treatment of skin irritation and application of Lyclear according to the Resident Handbook and The Cedars Policy.
* recreational activities.

Figure 16.4: The Cedars aromatherapy consent form

CASE STUDY

The following case study is an example of the effect of aromatherapy on one resident's health outcomes:

History

The resident was admitted to The Cedars in June 1996 because she was unable to manage the normal activities of daily living unaided, continually wandered, had disturbed sleep and short term memory loss. Information gained from the family revealed that her condition had deteriorated steadily over the preceding six months, and her husband was also developing the signs and symptoms of dementia. On admission to The Cedars she was 85 years old and had congestive cardiac failure and Alzhiemer's disease. Her medications at that time were Melleril 10 mg noctè, Lasix, 40 mg manè and

KCL 60 mgs mane. During the next three months Hemineurin 1 BD and Serenace 1.5 mg BD were added.

It was apparent that the addition of these medications did not assist in reducing her dementia behaviours. Adverse reactions were noted and the Melleril and Hemineurin were ceased and the Serenace was slowly reduced over twelve months. Her medications at the time of writing this chapter were, Serenace 1.5 mgs on alternate days, and Panamax 500 mgs TDS.

Despite these changes she still wandered aimlessly and frequently exhibited disturbed sleep. Members of the aromatherapy committee assessed her in 1999 after they received a referral from the staff stating that her sleep pattern was becoming increasingly disturbed and she was more restless and agitated. It was thought that some of the behavioural issues were exacerbated by lack of sleep. The committee commenced monitoring her sleep patterns and other behaviour. Following a detailed assessment the committee decided to implement an aromatherapy treatment plan which consisted of: lavender *(Lavendula angustifolia)*, 1 drop on her nightie and 1 drop on the pillow noctè, marjoram *(Origanum marjorana)*, 1 drop on her nightie and 1 drop on the pillow nocte.

Evaluation of therapy

Table 16.1 compares the number of sleep disturbance episodes before and after marjoram and lavender aromatherapy treatments were instituted. Figures 16.5 and 16.6 also depict her sleep disturbance before and after aromatherapy treatment. Sleep disturbance was defined as wandering, verbal disruption, resisting staff and irregular sleeping patterns. The number of sleep disturbance episodes were recorded on the data collection sheet every hour.

There was a 34% reduction in the number of sleep disturbance episodes for this lady, (see Figure 16.6). Clinical documentation during and immediately preceding the trial indicated that her episodes of aimless wandering, agitation and aggressive reactions to interventions decreased. If the program continues to be successful, the medical officer may withdraw the Serenace on a trial basis.

Similar trials have been conducted with other residents with comparable results. The Cedars is continuing to implement and monitor aromatherapy trials as part of the quality management program. It is anticipated that the data gathered from The Cedars and other facilities in the Northern Rivers region will contribute to establishing outcome-based research into aromatherapy.

Without marjoram and lavender		Marjoram and lavender applied	
Day	Sleep disturbance episodes	Day	Sleep disturbance episodes
1	0	1	0
2	0	2	0
3	1	3	0
4	1	4	0
5	6	5	1
6	2	6	0
7	4	7	0
8	7	8	4
9	1	9	1
10	1	10	0
11	1	11	2
12	4	12	2
13	4	13	1
14	0	14	0
Total 32		**Total 11**	

Table 16.1: Comparison of sleep disturbance before and after the application of marjoram and lavender

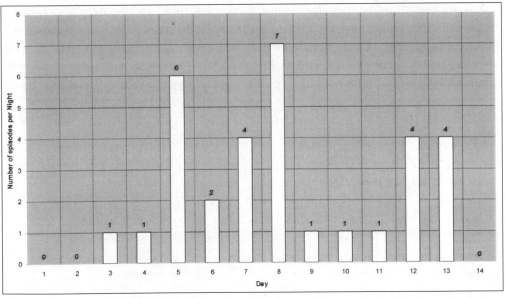

Figure 16.5: Record of sleep disturbance episodes before use of marjoram and lavender

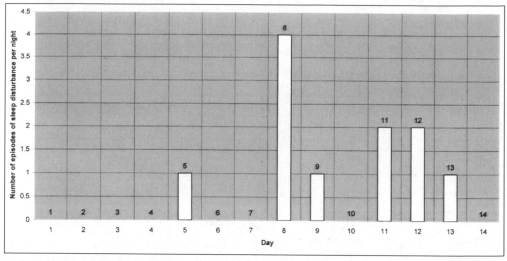

Figure 16.6: Record of sleep disturbance episodes after use of marjoram and lavender

SUMMARY

It is important for health care facilities to recognise the heterogenous nature of caring for older people. The emergence of complementary therapies in aged care facilities is having a decided impact on raising this awareness. The aromatherapy program at The Cedars demonstrates that there are beneficial complementary treatment approaches to the care of older people that either eliminate or markedly reduce the invasive nature of the biomedical model of care. For The Cedars, the program has resulted in many positive outcomes and the staff look forward to the future. More information about aromatherapy can be found in Chapter 9, and developing guidelines in Chapter 3.

ACKNOWLEDGMENTS

Special acknowledgment is made to The Cedars Aromatherapy Committee: Russell Smith, Kerry Houguet, Chris Kirk, and Elanor Nixon. Without their valuable knowledge and contribution, this chapter would not have been possible.

REFERENCES

Auer J Repin Y and Roe M (1993): *Just Change: The Cost Conscious Managers Tool Kit.* Australia: National Reference Centre for Continuing Education in Primary Health Care: University of Wollongong.

Bates L and Linder-Pelz S (1992): *Health Care Issues* (2nd edn). Sydney: Allen & Unwin.

Brown P (1994): *Health Care and the Aged, A nursing Perspective* (2nd edn). Artarmon: MacLennan & Petty Pty Limited.

Davis A. and George J (1993): *Health and Illness in Australia* (2nd edn). Australia: Harper Educational, p. 319.

Davis Judith A (1994): *Older Australians: A Positive View of Ageing.* Marrickville: Harcourt Brace & Company, p. 60.

Department of Health and Family Services (1997): *The Residential Care Manual.* Department of Health and Family Services. Canberra: AGPS.

Ewles L and Simnett I (1992): *Promoting Health: A Practical Guide* (2nd edn). Middlesex: Scutari Press.

Hartigan E (1978): Discharge planning: Identification of high risk groups. *Nursing Management* 18(12):30.

Howe A (ed.) (1985): *Towards an Older Australia.* Brisbane: University of Queensland Press.

Johnstone M-J (1995): *Bioethics: A Nursing Perspective.* Australia: Harcourt Brace and Company.

New South Wales Nurses Association (1999): *Legal and Professional Resource Kit for Nurses.* Sydney: New South Wales Nurses Association: 1.9 and 3.1.

New South Wales Nurses Association (1998): *Policy on Complementary Therapies in Nursing Practice.* Sydney: New South Wales Nurses Association.

Nurses Registration Board of New South Wales (1998): *Complementary Therapies in Nursing Practice.* Sydney: NRB New South Wales.

Rorden JW and Taft E (1990) *Discharge Planning Guide for Nurses.* Philadelphia: Harcourt Brace Jovanovich, Inc., p. 182.

Sax S (1990): *Health Care Choices and the Public Purse.* Sydney: Allen & Unwin Pty Ltd.

Sherman B (1991): *Dementia with Dignity: A Handbook for Carers.* Australia: McGraw-Hill Book Company Australia Pty Limited, p. 1.

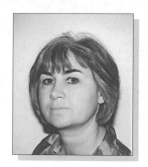

ROSE OSBORNE
Master in Primary Health Care, Therapeutic Touch, Diploma
of Professional Massage and Aromatherapy, Diploma of
Applied Science, RN, Diploma of Dental Therapy. Current
study: Doctor of Nursing, University of Adelaide

As a nurse–clinician with twelve years' experience in palliative care,
I currently combine clinical nursing responsibilities with teaching,
research and postgraduate studies, demonstrating depth and
commitment to clinical nursing practice. With additional
qualifications in professional massage and aromatherapy, I work
passionately towards the promotion of a non-institutional
environment, and the integration of various therapeutic
interventions not commonly used within the current medical and
nursing model of care. By working to improve the quality of life of
dying persons and their carers, I am developing personally as I learn
more about the human experience.

Chapter 17

Complementary therapies in a palliative care setting: the clinical experience

INTRODUCTION

Palliative care has evolved as a specialised area of health care. In palliative care, the importance of attending to the psychological, social, cultural and spiritual needs of the person as well as the physical aspects of care is acknowledged, in order to aid and support them until death and beyond (bereavement phase).

Daw House Hospice, opened in 1988, is a free standing, 15-bed hospice unit which services patients in need of palliative care in the southern area of Adelaide, South Australia. Here, the broad aims of care are centred on providing comfort to dying persons, their family and friends. Care in this context includes working towards relieving distress, supporting each patient's existing vitality and raising their spirits, that is, improving outlook and mood. Family and friends are welcomed into the environment and are encouraged to be actively involved in the care of their loved ones.

It is against a background of increasing public interest in broadening the scope of health care and enhancing the quality of available life that complementary approaches have become an integral part of service provision in this palliative care setting over the last decade. 'Complementary' in this context embodies the idea of coexistence and enhancement and can be defined as 'two or more things mutually complementing each other's deficiencies' (Rankin-Box, 1988:5). Nurses take a leading role in complementary care at Daw House Hospice. They contribute positively by creating a harmonious environment. The original clinical hospital environment has been transformed into a homely, calming atmosphere. Nurses, by virtue of their round-the-clock presence and unique working relationship with the environment, have taken a lead in the transformation.

Nurses also incorporate complementary care philosophy into their health care practice. In this environment, there is a willingness to acknowledge and promote the use of a wide range of interventions, both conventional and complementary, in nursing practice. Selected complementary therapies have been systematically incorporated into nursing care as they fit with the Simms (1986) classification. Therapies are judged suitable for palliative care under this classification if they are potentially comfort promoting, relatively non-invasive, easily understood by patient and practitioner, and affordable. There is also growing evidence that these therapies can have a positive effect on quality of life.

Consistent and persistent focus on complementary care at Daw House Hospice has been a powerful tool in hardening what used to be seen as 'soft options', thereby closing the gap between orthodox and non-orthodox health care. The new model of care is consistent with Brooks (1997:3):

> *Complementary in this context strives to mean complementary to the person, not necessarily the science of medicine and complementary with the person. It is therefore the provision of a choice of care that at its core, offers and finds resonance with the person for whom it is intended and by whom it is used.*

SUMMARY OF CONTENTS

This chapter examines the integration of complementary therapies into the model of care in a palliative care setting in South Australia. It is divided into four parts that together describe a process for advancing complementary care.

Part 1: Establishing a complementary care centre
The establishment of a complementary care centre and a program of complementary care as a nursing initiative is examined. Through this program, dying patients and their carers are given access to health care options that are not commonly offered in a hospital environment.

Part 2: Changing attitudes towards complementary care
Nurses in this palliative care setting are respected for their ability to care for patients and have the clinical freedom to express their healing instincts in an individual and

creative manner. Professional issues surrounding this increased scope of nursing practice are examined in order to promote and ensure safe, competent and compassionate nursing care.

Part 3: Integration of complementary therapies into nursing care: an example
Complementary nursing interventions are creatively combined with conventional medical treatments for common symptoms in the dying patient. In the example, aromatic hot towel compress and abdominal massage are used to complement traditional means of promoting bowel comfort. There is a focus on the physiological processes to promote bowel comfort, as well as an exploration of the domain of awareness and consciousness of both the nurse and patient.

Part 4: Evaluating complementary care
An evaluative research project, funded by a medical research grant, provides the opportunity to examine how the inclusion of a range of therapies into the provision of palliative care actually influences health behaviours and health status of dying patients and their carers.

PART 1: ESTABLISHING A COMPLEMENTARY CARE CENTRE

A complementary care centre ('the Centre') was established at Daw House Hospice in January 1995 to draw together existing resources, knowledge and skills relating to the use of complementary therapies in palliative care, and to formulate future directions for their place within the work of the Southern Community Hospice Program (SCHP).

In this innovative program, patients, carers and staff have access to health care options that are not commonly experienced in a hospital environment. Activities at the Centre are designed to enhance existing palliative care services by providing complementary therapies to patients and carers in an attempt to improve their quality of life during the dying process. As a nursing initiative, the Centre, coordinated by a registered nurse with qualifications in counselling and professional massage, is supported by the participation of volunteers with professional knowledge and skills related to selected complementary therapies. The Centre aims to:
* provide a peaceful place for patients, their carers and staff of the SCHP to visit, where physical, social, emotional and spiritual needs are acknowledged
* provide an operational base for selected complementary therapies
* encourage, and enable self-responsibility for dying patients, their carers and the Centre's staff

- establish a program of education, staff development and support
- research the impact of the program and selected therapies on patients' quality of life.

PART 2: CHANGING ATTITUDES TO COMPLEMENTARY CARE

The vision, leadership and clear directions that are provided at the clinical nurse level at Daw House Hospice have been vital in the integration of complementary therapies into nursing care. A number of influencing factors have led to increased acceptance of various therapies in this palliative care setting.

1. Supportive environment
Initial patronising attitudes have shifted over the years. Nurses are encouraged and supported by other members of the team to be creative in their care, provided there is theoretical underpinning for the selected complementary therapies. Nurses are also more supportive of their peers. There is increased recognition of the need to provide the necessary 'time out' to enable interested nurses to be involved with patients in these intensive care sessions.

2. Accessing financial resources
Donations are made to Daw House Hospice by relatives and patients in response to the intensive care received. Traditionally, nurses are not skilled at extracting money from the health care system. A coordinated complementary care program is crucial to the provision of quality palliative care, as patient's perceptions indicate. Small research grants and other money have been accessed to fund the activities described in Parts 1 and 2. However, vigorous promotion resulting in reliable funding will validate the use of complementary therapies and ensure that complementary care continues as an important, integral aspect of palliative nursing care.

3. Promoting the value of expert knowledge and skills
Patients are encouraged and supported in their choice of therapies and practitioners. The use of independent complementary practitioners is encouraged as a valid option, but dying patients are often unable to keep appointments. Nurses with expert knowledge and skills related to various therapeutic interventions are in an ideal position to provide these treatment options.

Nurses working at Daw House Hospice have sought additional credentials in therapies such as counselling, massage, aromatherapy, and energetic healing methods including reiki, therapeutic touch and touch for health. Although therapies such as massage and aromatherapy can be easily integrated into nursing care, suitably qualified persons are needed in each area to guide knowledge and skill development and to ensure safe, effective and appropriate practice.

4. Policy development

The process of integration, and the development of relevant and workable policies relating to complementary care within the SCHP has been a rather haphazard process. While recognising the need for policies to reflect the rights of patients and ensure professional standards, it has also been important that professionals are not regulated so inflexibly that an important opportunity to advance practice is lost.

Nurses at Daw House have moved from practice that is rule governed, as in Benner's (1984) description of the novice and advanced beginner. What is encouraged requires the development of perceptual awareness, clinical knowledge and experience that leads to proficient expert practice. Practical guidelines have been developed that are principle based rather than regulatory. They are designed to reflect the need for a safe, ethical and professional standard of care. Informed patient consent, confidentiality and the need to document are central constructs in these guidelines. Staff education on central issues is an integral part of nursing practice.

While the development of national policies is seen as a necessary step towards safe standards of care and will help to validate the use of various complementary therapies in nursing practice, nurses do not have time to 're-invent the wheel'. The advantage that nurses at Daw House Hospice have is an integrated model of nursing care in action, which is being used as a reference by other nursing institutions. More information about developing guidelines and policies can be found in Chapter 3.

PART 3: INTEGRATION OF COMPLEMENTARY THERAPIES INTO NURSING CARE

The method used to integrate complementary therapies into nursing care is shown using the example of an aromatic hot towel compress and abdominal massage for abdominal discomfort and constipation. In palliative care, digestive disorders and bowel dysfunction, particularly constipation, are common, uncontrolled symptoms. Contributing factors include decreased mobility, reduced food and fluid intake, wasting and weakness of the abdominal muscles, anxiety and other emotional overload, increased pharmacological intervention (notably narcotics) and/or disease process involving the alimentary tract.

In the treatment of gastric upset and constipation, a whole spectrum of medical and non-medical therapeutically equivalent options are known to be available. An aromatic hot towel treatment together with abdominal massage can be used with various conventional medical interventions such as enemas, suppositories and oral aperients. Aromatic hot towel compress can be used alone, or prior to abdominal massage. Both are effective treatments for digestive disorders, including gastric upset and decreased alimentary tract motility from mild to severe constipation. Chaitow (1999:2) states that treatments such as the application of hot and cold compresses 'are so dramatically effective, so simple to apply, and so safe.'

Hot compress as part of modern hydrotherapy, together with the therapeutic use of aromas and touch, are great examples of folk medicine being brought up to date. The application of damp heat to an area leads to an increased circulation in that region, followed by increased metabolic activity involving the whole body, including tissue relaxation and reduction of pain and spasm. A hot towel compress combined with aromatic abdominal massage enables selected essential oils to be in contact with the large area of the skin and underlying muscles of the abdominal area. Essential oils that have a particular therapeutic effect on the digestive system include antispasmodics. These quickly relax any nervous tension that may be causing digestive spasm or colic. Examples include clary sage (*Salvia sclarea*), ginger (*Zingiber officinalis*) and peppermint (*Mentha piperita*). Carminatives also affect the digestive system by relaxing the stomach muscles, increasing the peristalsis of the intestine and reducing the production of gas in the system. Examples include black pepper (*Piper nigrum*), rosemary (*Rosmarinus officinalis*), clary sage (*Salvia sclarea*) and peppermint (*Mentha piperita*) (Battaglia, 1995:405–406).

In the example given here, nurses operate within a high degree of personal and professional accountability. Instead of relying on a narrow conceptual nursing model, clinical decisions are justified from the nurse's assessment of individual patients in specific situations. Accountability begins with the decision to treat the patient. Such an offer is made in full consultation with medical, nursing and any other relevant team members. Informed consent is an integral part of treatment. Nurses are instructed in the basic principles of abdominal massage, aromatherapy and hot towel compresses. Safe practice is emphasised (see Table 17.1).

Nurses are responsible for ensuring that the procedure is fully described to the patient and family. All aspects of the procedure are documented, including the selection of essential oil (or oils), patient's and nurse's reflections about the treatment, and the effect on bowel comfort, including bowel motion. Throughout the procedure, the nurse

Preparing the environment

1. Ensure area is warm, comfortable, and private and eliminate the possibility of interruptions.
2. Organise equipment, including adjusting the bed height and access to a commode chair.
3. Select music in consultation with patient if appropriate.
4. Take time to centre, as a disciplined way to slow down and clear distractions.
5. Encourage patient to centre and focus on the treatment.

Aromatic hot towel treatment

1. Select essential oil/s according to the symptoms.
2. Prepare hot towel solution by combining:
   - 5 drops of selected essential oil/s
   - 5 mls of emulsifier (e.g. full cream milk)
   - 750 mls of hot water (47 degrees centigrade)
3. Pour the solution over a hand towel or small bath towel.
4. Squeeze out excess moisture and check with patient that the temperature is comfortable.
5. Place hot towel over the abdominal area and cover the area with plastic sheet to retain heat.
6. Remain with the patient, encouraging patient to remain centered.
7. Remove compress after five minutes.

Aromatic abdominal massage (Battaglia, 1995:28)

1. Prepare massage oil (1% solution) by combining
   - 20 mls of carrier oil (e.g. almond oil)
   - 4 drops of selected essential oil/s.
2. Apply the oil blend liberally to the abdominal area so as not to create a pulling effect on the delicate abdominal tissue.
3. Massage in a clockwise direction following the direction of the alimentary tract from the ascending colon, across the transverse colon and down the descending colon.
4. Massage gently at first then gradually working deeper according to the patient's tolerance.
5. For maximum effect continue for 10–15 minutes as tolerated.

Documentation

1. Document procedure, including selected essential oil/s, procedural perceptions (patient and nurse) and results (including any effect on bowel comfort or function).
2. Discuss relevant aspects of the procedure with other members of the team as necessary.

Warning:

Abdominal massage is not recommended if bowel obstruction is evident or suspected. Discontinue the procedure if patient reports or appears to be uncomfortable or unwilling to continue.

Table 17.1: Procedural guidelines for aromatic hot towel compress and abdominal massage

needs to work with intuition, sensitive hands and a compassionate heart. Some internal preparation is therefore required. Before beginning the intervention it is important that both nurse and patient take the opportunity to centre—that is to quiet and clear the self, to get in touch with the inner self, and to reach peacefulness. Breath awareness is an excellent way to reach this state. Clinical nursing practice in this instance becomes a blend of empirical, pragmatic, intuitive, and artistic nursing care that emphasises safe practice and therapeutic effect.

PART 4: EVALUATING COMPLEMENTARY CARE

The advancement of complementary care will rest considerably upon the evidence of nursing research. Cognisant of this fact, a research project entitled, 'Evaluation of complementary therapies in a palliative care setting', was undertaken to examine how the inclusion of a range of complementary therapies in the provision of palliative care actually influences health behaviours and the health status of the consumers. The project was funded by the JH and JD Gunn Medical Research Foundation.

The project did not attempt to examine the effectiveness of individual therapies, but focused on personal perceptions of a series of three visits to the Centre. Participants were recruited from patients, carers and staff of the Southern Community Hospice Program including nine community patients, five in-patients, three principal carers and three staff.

The researchers examined the contextual explanations that this qualitative approach produced to increase understanding about the issues and concerns of dying patients and their carers. The information gained was used to assist patients to live fully, not just survive, and to assist with the ongoing development of the complementary care program (Osborne et al., 1997:21–26).

Constraints experienced in conducting research in the palliative care setting
Determining the effects and the clinical significance of the complementary interventions was difficult because:
- three people died without completing the study
- the subject population was very frail and their ability to participate was extremely unpredictable
- some subjects experienced the rapid changes in physical and emotional status that are part of the terminal phase of illness
- benefits were often overshadowed by deterioration in other ways

- the type of outcome chosen, i.e. seeking insight into perceived benefits, is not easily quantifiable.

Despite these constraints some significant findings were identified.

Relief of symptoms

Anecdotal evidence from this study suggests that access to the complementary care service can improve the quality of life for people in their final stages of life. Total relaxation and relief of symptoms, however, is a very difficult state for dying patients and carers to achieve. Grief, serious illness, physical and emotional trauma and extreme relationship reorganisation are major issues engulfing the dying person.

Development of a therapeutic relationship

Participants consistently described interactions and the development of relationships. They placed great value on simple things such as kindness and uncomplicated 'humanness'. These attributes:

> ... *have commonality in all human beings and all human culture and across time, are the things that touch our hearts, which make us feel loved, which make us become more aware of ourselves.*

> (Reilly, 1995:25).

A therapeutic relationship is one of the most important aspects of medical care. Reilly (1995:25) describes a therapeutic relationship thus:

> ... *the question of intention and integrity; the quality of the meeting; the trust; the relationship; the shared walk together of the person and the carer is where the magic really happens, where things really move and people experience radical changes in how they are coping or not coping, and in the quality of their life, and where transformations occur.*

An effective consultation can unfold, feelings can be expressed and trust may be established when you are with someone and you talk with them and listen to their response. A healing encounter occurs when you bring some simple, positive intervention to the situation. One nurse explored her concept of a healing encounter:

> *We exchange greetings—a few words of kindness. We hold hands and sit together as human beings with feelings, experiences and needs. We sense giving and receiving love and attention and time; the intensity of the encounter, the*

tears; the experience of a sudden release of memories; the smells and the touch. This is all 'therapy'. The product of all this is growing and learning.

(Osborne, 1999).

Therapeutic environment

One of the principle aims of the Centre is to provide a quiet peaceful place for people to visit. There is little doubt that the physical environment can positively affect therapeutic outcomes. When participants visited the Centre, they frequently commented on the homely décor and the subtle but evocative aromas and music which all help to create a relaxed, non-institutionalised peaceful place. The pace is unhurried and participants felt that someone who was prepared to listen to their fears and concerns gave them individual time and attention.

When you are in a healing environment, you know it; no analysis is required. You should somehow feel welcome, balanced and at one with yourself and the world. You are both relaxed and stimulated, reassured and invited to expand. You feel at home.

(Venolia, 1988:33).

Individual growth and learning

All participants indicated they were undergoing considerable personal growth. They welcomed the opportunity to reflect and address feelings and issues about loss and grief and their personal coping abilities. Participants were encouraged to initiate contact with the service and some felt this contributed to their feelings of having choice and control over their care options. The nurses gained confidence in complementary care as a valuable option for patients and carers, and everybody expressed high motivation to continue their involvement with the service.

One of the aims of the Centre is to acknowledge the practitioners' own health needs. Nurses and volunteers reported personal and professional growth, with the expansion of their roles in hospice care. Nurses appreciated fewer time constraints and the changes in the priority given to clinical interventions and procedures. Involvement in the service has enhanced their emotional wellbeing by providing an opportunity to resolve personal issues about loss and grief.

Through their involvement, volunteers felt increased satisfaction as they gained new skills and knowledge that broadened their perceived ability to 'help'. Volunteers felt that the service was worthy of their time and work and represented an opportunity to grow and develop.

Implications of research

Anecdotal evidence from the evaluation suggests that the non-institutional environment, purposeful contact, individual therapy sessions and the development of a therapeutic relationship over the period of the study contributed to the patients' quality of life. All patients reported an increased sense of wellbeing and feelings that the contact was valuable. Although current financial difficulties have resulted in a reduction in the activities of the Centre, evidence gained from this evaluation has encouraged us to creatively explore funding options for coordination and service delivery as well as to work to improve the design and effectiveness of the service.

CONCLUSIONS: BEYOND COMPLEMENTARY

Nurses at Daw House Hospice are taking a leading role in raising consumer awareness about complementary care and increasing the diversity of choices in health care. Advocating the incorporation of appropriate complementary therapies into health care plans will mean that these therapies will eventually be integral to health care. As such, the interventions will not need to be referred to as 'complementary' and will be available in all areas of care, not only palliative care.

By blending conventional with non-conventional interventions nurses can be actively involved in renewing and enhancing the art of nursing. The use of interventions such as aromatic hot towel treatments and abdominal massage integrated into daily nursing care will augment nursing care and offer patients more choice and nurses more variety, thereby adding new dimensions to existing health care. Clinical nursing practice in this instance is a blend of the empirical, pragmatic, intuitive and artistic, with the emphasis on safe practice and therapeutic effect.

REFERENCES

Battaglia S (1995): *The Complete Guide to Aromatherapy.* Virginia Qld: The Perfect Potion.

Benner P (1984): *From Novice to Expert.* Menlo Park: Addison-Wesley.

Brooks P (1997): The complementary care connections. Paper presented at the Complementary Care Seminar, Repatriation General Hospital, May 1997.

Chaitow L (1999): *Water Therapy for Health and Beauty.* Shaftesbury, Dorset: Element Books Limited.

Osborne R, Parker D, Maddocks I (1997): Evaluation of Complementary Therapies in a Palliative Care Setting. International Institute of Hospice Studies: pp.21–26 (unpublished report).

Rankin-Box D (1988): *Complementary Therapies in Nursing.* Sydney: Croom Helm.

Reilly D (1995): Research, homeopathy and the therapeutic consultation. *Alternative Therapies* Sept 1(4).

Simms S (1986): Slow stroke back massage for cancer patients. *Nursing Times* 83:28–29.

Venolia C (1988): *Healing Environments.* Berkeley, CA: Celestial Arts.

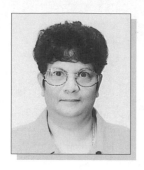

SUSIE NANAYAKKARA
RN (UK), RM (UK), Diploma of Plastic Surgery (UK), Diploma of Aromatherapy (Australia)

Clinical Nurse Specialist, Auburn Hospital, NSW

Susie trained in England and has wide clinical nursing experience gained overseas and in Australia. She worked as a senior midwife at Royal Berkshire Hospital, Reading, before coming to Australia in 1989. Since then she has been working as a clinical nurse specialist at Auburn Hospital. Susie has always been interested in complementary therapies and completed a Diploma of Aromatherapy in 1991. She is co-author of a book on baby massage published in 1996. Susie won the Auburn Hospital and Community Health Services International Nurses' Day award in 1998 for her contribution and commitment to improving patient care. At present she is involved in conducting workshops on female genital mutilation (FGM) and is a member of the team assisting in the formulation of a self-directed learning package for counsellors and a training manual for health workers.

Complementary therapies in midwifery practice

Childbirth is a natural process and midwifery is the art or practice of assisting women in all aspects of the birthing process. One of the major aspects of midwifery care is supporting women in dealing with the pain of labour in line with their expectations. Despite this, in the past, there has been minimal interest in, and few options for, drug-free pain relief in the traditional hospital setting, although the midwifery literature has provided support for such options in recent years (Rankin-Box, 1995; Yerby, 1996; and Liburd, 1999).

THE CHALLENGE FOR CHANGE

In the early 1990s the maternity staff at Auburn Hospital started examining their role in offering women alternative mechanisms for coping during labour. An impetus to change was the Ministerial Task Force Report on Obstetric Services in New South Wales. Since the 1980s women have become more informed and consequently more vocal in their demand for increased choice of care in pregnancy and childbirth. The report highlighted this and recommended recognition of differing cultural preferences in childbirth, the encouragement of non-medicated pain relief and the provision of a more homelike atmosphere (Ministerial Task Force on Obstetric Services in New South Wales 1989).

The clientele using Auburn Hospital's maternity services come from a range of cultural backgrounds—including all parts of Asia, Africa and the Middle East—and are heavily influenced in childbirth decisions by family and tradition. This frequently results in women not wanting pain during labour but, at the same time, refusing medicated pain relief. The conventional pain relief options are narcotic injection, epidural anaesthesia and/or inhalation analgesia. Midwives were encouraging ambulation and positioning to achieve comfort but these measures were not always culturally acceptable. Massage was limited to an occasional rub on the 'sore spot'.

In the early 1990s, renovations had already taken place to create a less clinical environment and attitudes were a lot less prescriptive in care management. The birth unit was freshly painted in pastel colours and each room was provided with an ensuite. The effect was welcoming and very different from the traditional hospital environment. The author, who had read about and become interested in aromatherapy, suggested that this complementary therapy could be useful for relaxation and possibly beneficial in relieving pain. Shirley Price (1993:255) certainly made it sound like the answer in her definition of aromatherapy:

> ... *the controlled use of essential oils to maintain and promote the health and vitality of the spirit, the emotions and the physical body. This incorporates many practical methods of application, such as inhalation, baths, compresses, self-application and massage.*

The idea gained the support of the staff because of the potential advantages to the women:

- It offered increased choice of pain relief with minimal risk for mother and baby.
- It was not mistrusted as an intervention.
- It helped make the environment less clinical.
- It would increase interaction between the midwife and the woman.
- It would mean no delay because it would be midwife initiated.
- It would clear minds for decision making.
- It would mean that women could retain their ability to engage in activities that promote labour progress.
- It would smell nice.

To lend credence to the use of aromatherapy for pain relief we needed a sound knowledge base and a qualified aromatherapist. The author was sponsored by the hospital to attend the Re Nu College and acquired a Diploma of Aromatherapy. A series of workshops was then set up to educate the maternity staff. The midwives learnt different forms of massage and the appropriate use of various essential oils. Hydrotherapy was not popular in midwifery at the time and the topic wasn't included in the workshops. The concept, however, was familiar from general nursing practice and the advantages to midwifery were soon recognised.

INTRODUCING AROMATHERAPY

The formalised support from the hospital executive, the enthusiasm generated by the workshops and the encouragement of a few staunch midwife and medical officer supporters did much to facilitate the introduction of aromatherapy. Many of the staff and clientele were quick converts and there was never any strong opposition to using aromatherapy. It is possible some people didn't object because they didn't consider aromatherapy to be a true therapy. Others may have regarded it as just another trendy fashion.

Aromatherapy was introduced quietly, one step at a time. Fresh fragrances, in a water-based spray, frequently wafted along the corridors of the birth unit, and staff and clients alike rejoiced in the interesting aromas that replaced the traditional hospital smell of disinfectant. An oil vapouriser was placed out of sight in the office of the director of nursing and the resulting relaxation led to approval for the use of aromatherapy and funding for essential oils and equipment. The clientele were seduced by the aromas during open days, birth unit tours and in the antenatal clinic. This gentle introduction was important as women and staff alike learned which aromas were pleasing and, just as importantly, those which were not. Doctors and midwives alike readily accepted most aromas but there were two essential oils that caused some difficulties. Some found jasmine (*Jasminum officinale*) sickly sweet, and rose geranium (*Pelargonium graveolens*) too pungent. One doctor also claimed that rose geranium gave him a headache.

Most women seem to enjoy an aroma even if it has no therapeutic value, so the use of a light fragrance in the delivery rooms created a welcoming environment. The positive reaction to establishing a pleasant aroma was apparent when the women seemed to relax more quickly (Burns, 1992; and, Walsh and Morrissey, 1998). Initially the fragrance was diffused into the air through jars made of porous clay but later electric oil vapourisers were introduced as a safe and more effective alternative.

TYPES OF OILS USED

There are two types of oils used—essential oils and carrier oils.

Essential oils
These are called the 'living force' or 'energy source' of the plant kingdom. They are reputed to influence mood, being either enlivening or sedating. Essential oils have been found to have various properties experimentally and clinically (Valnet, 1982), for example, antiviral, antibacterial, antifungal, antiseptic, anti-inflammatory, sedative,

analgesic and stimulating to the movement of body fluids. Essential oils are highly flammable and volatile, evaporating rapidly to form vapours. When exposed to air, some oils will oxidise. Essential oils should be used externally only and never undiluted. It is the policy of Auburn Hospital that essential oils are the only ingredient that should be added to a carrier oil. It is wise never to use synthetic oil mixes because they will not be effective in achieving the therapeutic outcome desired (Valnet, 1982).

Some of the essential oils that have been found useful in our midwifery practice at Auburn are listed below.

*   Eucalyptus *(Eucalyptus globulus)* is antibacterial, decongestant and energising. Though used for its decongestant properties it is often chosen for its aroma alone.
*   Jasmine *(Jasminum officinale)* contains many of the properties of rose (see below) but it is expensive and it overwhelms some people. Jasmine is not recommended for use during pregnancy, but is suitable to use during labour.
*   Lavender *(Lavandula officinalis)* is antidepressant, soothing, calming and balancing. This oil has proven to be the most popular and is used for relaxation by either massage or inhalation.
*   Lemon *(Citrus limon)* and grapefruit *(Citrus paradisi)* are uplifting and refreshing. A few drops in water may be sprayed as an air freshener.
*   Peppermint *(Mentha piperita)* is analgesic, decongestant and antispasmodic. It has been found to be useful for nausea associated with labour (Tiran, 1996).
*   Rose *(Rosa centifolia)* is uplifting and a hormone balancer. Because of its antidepressant qualities it has been very useful for women who have had an intrauterine death.
*   Rose geranium *(Pelargonium graveolens)* is antidepressant, uplifting and a hormone balancer. Although reputed to be useful for postnatal depression it can also be used as an alternative to rose or lavender, according to a woman's preference.
*   Sandalwood *(Santalum album)* is relaxing, sedating and warming. It is beneficial in preserving the aroma in essential oil blends.

Tisserand (1977) and Arcier (1992) have described in detail the properties of the oils listed above as well as other essential oils that have uses in midwifery. Some of these other oils are:

*   Chamomile (Roman) *(Anthemis nobilis)* — calming, soothing, anti-inflammatory and very gentle oil for use during postnatal breast care.
*   Cypress *(Cupressus sempervirens)* — an astringent and good for treating haemorrhoids after delivery.
*   Sweet fennel *(Foeniculum vulgare)* — a hormone balancer that stimulates lactation.

Carrier oils

These are oils into which the essential oils are blended. They inhibit evaporation of the essential oil and encourage its absorption into the skin. They are also known as base oils.

Carrier oils have emollient value and contain vitamins that are beneficial for the skin of the mother and/or baby. The carrier oils also assist the masseur's hands to slide smoothly and avoid damage to the skin of the person being massaged.

There are many different types of carrier oils. Good carrier oils are sweet almond, apricot kernel, peach kernel, grape seed, olive oil or corn oil. Peanut oil or blended oils should not be used. It is important to remember that carrier oils should always be cold pressed, which means there is no change in the composition of the oil during extraction, because no heat is involved in the process. They should be stored in glass (preferably amber) and in a cool environment, out of direct sunlight.

ADMINISTRATION

Aromatherapy is administered in the birth unit by inhalation, or in combination with massage or hydrotherapy (baths and compresses).

Massage

The multiple benefits of massage are fully discussed in Chapter 9. However, they can be summarised as:
* physical — through its mechanical, physiological and reflex effects
* emotional — through its effects via the sense of touch
* mental — by promoting a feeling of wellbeing
* spiritual/energy — through the interchange of energies between the patient and the practitioner.

INDICATIONS FOR AND METHOD OF MASSAGE

Aromatherapy massage is used for the general effects described above, but more specifically for emotional support, easing of muscle tension, and natural pain relief through the release of endorphins. It lends itself especially to midwifery by:
* deepening the bond between midwife and woman
* providing natural pain relief
* easing muscle tension

- encouraging relaxation
- complementing a normal process
- relieving stress and tension related to childbirth and motherhood
- lessening common discomforts of pregnancy
- relieving minor discomforts for babies, e.g. gas and constipation.

A good massage oil can be made by adding essential oils to a carrier oil to achieve a 2.5% concentration e.g. to 20 millilitres of a carrier oil add eight drops of one essential oil and two drops of sandalwood. 10% of the carrier oil can consist of wheat germ oil to prevent oxidisation, because it contains vitamin E, a natural anti-oxidant. Essential oil blends at the Auburn hospital are prepared by the aromatherapist.

Massage oils should not be used where there is a history of skin allergies or skin disease. At Auburn it has not been the practice to use routine skin testing because the essential oil concentrations used are weak and the selection of oils is restricted to a few well known oils. No skin reactions have occurred. There is, however, a chance of unknown allergies and it would be safer to introduce skin testing (Tisserand and Balacs, 1995).

Oil is applied with a movement of effleurage (a gentle sliding movement that is soothing to the skin). Massage is commonly used for the benefit of both mother and baby.

Mother
- Helps relieve mothers of tension, backache, breast engorgement and the 'baby blues'.
- Tension: Although any massage seems to help tension, massaging the neck and shoulders is the most effective. Commence effleurage using the palms of the hands and start from the base of the shoulder blades and work up and around the shoulders. Petrissage (squeezing the muscles) is best used on the shoulders to release tension and toxins from the muscles. Use the hand and fingers to gently squeeze the shoulders working from the neck towards the arm. Circular movement over the Trapezius muscle helps to relieve upper back tension. Place the hands on either side of the spine and using circular movements of the thumbs work up the sides of the spine towards the neck. Foot massage is also an effective way to reduce the experience of pain (Hulme et al., 1999).
- Backache: Backache in the labouring woman is often caused by a posterior position of the fetus. A back massage while the woman is on all-fours (on hands and knees) is beneficial. Placing cushions and bean bags on the floor or bed for the woman to lean over may make the position more comfortable and easier to maintain. Apply the oil over the back area with gentle deep circular movements of the thumbs, working from the coccygeal area to the hip.

- Breast engorgement: Although breast engorgement is rarely seen these days, gentle massage of lumps and massage towards the nipple is effective in encouraging lymphatic drainage. Normally breast massage is not encouraged. Any essential oil used on the breasts should be washed off before feeding.
- 'Baby blues': Hormone changes may leave the woman feeling depressed. A full body massage can help her to relax and give her an increased sense of wellbeing. Some midwives say they themselves feel more relaxed after giving a woman a massage. Unfortunately time is often an issue in giving this sort of treatment but massage can easily be performed by the woman's partner or another member of her family.

Baby

The benefits of massage for the for the baby are:

- improvement in quality of sleep
- assistance in relaxation
- relief of colic, gas and constipation
- aid to positive nonverbal communication
- strengthening of respiratory and circulatory function
- encouraging weight gain in premature babies.

Newborn babies are massaged with carrier oils only, as essential oils are too concentrated (Turner and Nanayakkara, 1996). When massaging a baby it is important to use light pressure on the hands, legs and feet. All other areas are massaged with very light stroking movements.

Premature babies improve when they are gently stroked, showing weight gain and/or maturation. It is important to note, however, that some babies, such as those who are medically unstable, can be adversely affected by touch stimulation. Massage is frequently promoted for mother–child interaction and also keeps the mother calmer and makes her feel involved (Vickers, 1996).

Sessions in baby massage for parents are just being established and will be conducted by a midwife with a certificate in infant massage from the International Association of Infant Massage.

INHALATION

The sense of smell is the most evocative of all the senses as the olfactory system, the special sensory nerves of smell, quickly affects the limbic system where emotions are processed. Bad smelling substances are said to warn of danger, while great joy may come from a scented garden. Inhalation of the essential oils is the quickest, most direct route into the body due to the vapourisation and then the gaseous exchange in the lungs (Tisserand and Balacs, 1995).

Experience has shown that 'less is better' when using essential oils and two to five drops is all that is required. The aroma of the oil is effectively dispersed using an oil vapouriser, but a dish of hot water or a piece of cotton wool can also be used. The most common oils used for this purpose are peppermint for nausea, lavender for relaxation, rose for grieving, eucalyptus for congestion and floral and citrus oils for freshness.

HYDROTHERAPY

As with inhalation, compresses and baths require only a few drops of essential oil in the water. Water temperature should be tested on the inside of the wrist. Compresses are usually in the form of a well-wrung-out towel, nappy or sponge. Most women choose heat for comfort during labour although some prefer cool compresses to the perineum. There are several uses for hydrotherapy.

- Some women prefer a warm essential oil compress for the lower back or abdomen instead of a massage.
- Lavender compresses can be used to relieve the stinging sensation when the perineum is stretching to accommodate the baby's head during the second stage of labour.
- Sitz baths (a hip bath or a bowl large enough to sit in) are still popular with some people. Two drops of lavender oil in a bowl of water will help to sooth damaged tissue and encourage healing. Sitz baths also help to alleviate the discomfort of haemorrhoids.
- Essential oil mixed with water and sprayed on a face cloth and placed on the forehead is greatly appreciated by women, especially during summer months.
- During the second stage of labour some women prefer to have a face cloth soaked in lavender water over the forehead to relieve tension and keep them cool.
- Compresses can also be useful in easing the pain of breast engorgement.
- An essential oil bath is an effective alternative to body massage.
- Most women like their feet massaged or soaked in a bowl of water with a few drops of peppermint oil to soothe aches and pains.

AROMATHERAPY AND ANTENATAL EDUCATION

Aromatherapy is discussed in the antenatal period, either at classes or at a clinic visit, and women are encouraged to consider aromatherapy, both as an alternative to medicated pain relief and in conjunction with other forms of pain relief. Aromatherapy is popular with women as it supports labour and delivery as a natural process. They feel they are better able to give input into their treatment and care when drugs do not impede their judgement. However, the use of aromatherapy is not restricted to those who want a drug-free labour. It is often used in conjunction with heat, positioning, pelvic rocking and medicated pain relief if desired and appropriate. The antenatal discussions explain the effects of essential oils and also discourage women from experimenting. They also help women to choose their essential oil preferences, which are documented in their birth plan. The preparation of a birth plan encourages women to seek information about all aspects of childbirth, not only pain relief, and to realise that they have the right to give input into their care.

DOCUMENTATION AND EVALUATION

All therapies administered are documented and their effectiveness evaluated in the clinical records. Documentation in health care records should accurately and factually describe a patient's progress through an episode of care. This is important for providing effective communication between the health care team, facilitating effective continuing care and enabling evaluation of a patient's health outcomes. Documentation includes the practitioner's observations as well as the patient's statements concerning their own wellbeing. Good documentation is important for accurate evaluation. When aromatherapy is used, the indication for use, the type of oil used and the method of administration should be noted. Evaluation of effectiveness should reflect the reason for administration, although other effects/side effects should also be included.

SHARING THE CARING EXPERIENCE

The following examples indicate the success of using aromatherapy in maternity care.

Jasmine
Jasmine, a shy young girl of 16 years, was admitted to the birth unit in labour. She was very nervous and frightened as it was her first pregnancy. She had just arrived in Australia and could not speak English. With the aid of an interpreter, verbal consent was

obtained to the use of aromatherapy. Examination revealed Jasmine was only in early labour. Ambulation and warm showers were encouraged but she remained distressed.

The midwife commenced massaging Jasmine's hands and then feet with a blend of lavender and olive oil and could feel the stiffness going out of Jasmine's muscles. The midwife then massaged her back, shoulders and neck. After about 20 minutes Jasmine was obviously coping with the contractions even though they were becoming much stronger. Intermittent massage and showers were continued and she progressed without incident or analgesia to have a normal delivery of a beautiful 3.5kg baby girl.

Carol

Carol was in labour for the third time. Her first three labours were fairly easy as far as pain was concerned but nausea was a problem from the onset of regular contractions. Carol agreed to try aromatherapy. Three drops of peppermint oil were placed in a vapouriser soon after her arrival. There were no episodes of nausea throughout her labour.

Fatima

Fatima presented looking very distressed and was very oedemateous. Her blood pressure was 160/105 mm/Hg. While waiting for a medical officer to review Fatima, the midwife began a relaxing foot massage with lavender and sandalwood to try and calm her. When the medical officer arrived ten minutes later Fatima's blood pressure was 140/90 mm/Hg. The blood pressure was carefully monitored during labour, but no medical intervention was required. Aromatherapy massage was continued intermittently throughout labour.

DEVELOPING A POLICY

Policies are necessary for any institutions that use complementary therapies or treat patients who use complementary therapies themselves. The unit policy developed at Auburn Hospital is simple but prescriptive to ensure safety because there was no documented evidence that aromatherapy had ever been used in the hospital environment, certainly not in Australia, at the time the project commenced. There is now much more interest in and information about complementary therapies and a more comprehensive policy is being developed. The current policy was formulated by midwives and approved by medical officers. It includes the following as main points:
*   Blending of oils is to be performed by a qualified therapist.
*   All oils must be of good quality and not previously diluted or synthetic.
*   Either olive or sweet almond oil carrier oils are to be used.

- Essential oils are the only ingredient to be added to the carrier oil.
- Essential oils may be administered through vapourisers, hydrotherapy or massage.
- Verbal consent from the client is to be documented in the clinical notes.
- The indications for use, type of therapy used and evaluation of effectiveness are to be documented in the clinical record.

All midwives may practise aromatherapy within the limitations set by the policy. These limits reflect the level of education provided in the in-service training and have resulted in an excellent safety record (Price, 1998). More information about developing policies can be found in Chapter 3.

NINE YEARS LATER

The use of aromatherapy in the birth unit is monitored like any other treatment. Audits of documentation occur yearly and include the effectiveness of care given. Patient satisfaction surveys include satisfaction with pain relief offered. No criticism or adverse outcomes have been reported since aromatherapy was introduced. Some of the benefits expressed by families are that they feel more at home and in a relaxed atmosphere without the clinical hospital smells; they are able to adopt a more normal family supportive role; and they feel involved in the care instead of standing back.

Aromatherapy and massage help return some control of the labour process to the woman and her family, control which has been overly relinquished in the medical model of childbirth (Shore, 1998). The benefits expressed by the women include a feeling that something special/extra has been done for them and through the improved communication by touch they feel they are really being heard. Many have achieved a non-medicated labour, some planned, some unplanned. The midwives have witnessed a decrease in the use of narcotics and have developed a more inclusive role with the families. A demand has obviously been created as many requests for information and inservice education have been received from other hospitals. To date all requests have been granted. Aromatherapy also seems to be a therapy which crosses cultural boundaries, perhaps because it blends with healing concepts such as harmony and balance often found in folk healing traditions (Wing, 1998).

Formal evaluation of aromatherapy has been difficult due to other factors that influenced the outcomes and reflect some of the difficulties other authors have found in evaluating complementary therapies (Hobbs and Davies, 1998; and Botting and Cook, 1998). (More information about researching complementary therapies can be found in

Chapter 6.) Among the difficulties are the changing attitudes of midwives towards pain relief and interventions generally, the combination of activities used in conjunction with aromatherapy and the increased participation of the women in the planning of their care. Aromatherapy does create an environment that is conducive to relaxation and normality, which affects the staff, the women and their families. At the very least it makes the women feel pampered and, if the desired effect is achieved, women meet their expectations of a drug-free labour. After all, it must be more pleasant to have a baby born in a cabbage rose patch than in a cabbage patch.

ACKNOWLEDGMENTS

The author wishes to thank Auburn Hospital and Community Health Services for all the support and sponsorship which helped to initiate aromatherapy. Many thanks to Cecile Coughlin and Gladwyn Williams for all the encouragement, support and help afforded to me during this project. A special thanks to Roma and Phil Turner and to my co-workers without whose support and encouragement none of this would have been possible.

REFERENCES

Arcier M (1992): *Aromatherapy*. London: Hamlyn.

Botting D, Cook R (1998): Therapy evaluation: Evaluating the effectiveness of complementary therapies. *International Journal of Palliative Nursing* 4(1):32–6.

Burns E (1992): Dedicated to better birth. *The International Journal of Aromatherapy* 4(1):9–12.

Hobbs S, Davies PD (1998): Critical review of how nurses research massage therapy: are they using the best methods? *Complementary Therapies in Nursing and Midwifery* 4(2):35–40.

Hulme J, Waterman H, Hillier VF (1999): The effect of foot massage on patients. *Journal of Advanced Nursing* 30(2):460–8

Liburd A (1999): The use of complementary therapies in midwifery in the U.K. *Journal of Nurse Midwifery* 44(3):325-9, 183-188.

Ministerial Task Force Report on Obstetric Services in New South Wales (1989): *Maternity Services in New South Wales.* Sydney: NSW Department of Health.

Price S (1993): *Aromatherapy Workbook.* London: Thorsons, p.255.

Rankin-Box D (ed) (1995): *The Nurses' Handbook of Complementary Therapies.* Edinburgh: Churchill Livingstone.

Shore N (1998): The second stage of labour—who controls it? *Assignment* 4(1):20-5.

Tiran D (1996): Book of the month. Complementary therapies for nausea in pregnancy. *Modern-Midwife* 6(3):19-21.

Tisserand RB (1977): *The Art of Aromatherapy.* Saffron Walden, Essex: CW Daniel.

Tisserand R, Balacs T (1995): *Essential Oil Safety: A Guide for Health Professionals.* Edinburgh: Churchill Livingstone.

Turner R, Nanayakkara S (1996): *The Soothing Art of Baby Massage.* Sydney: Lansdowne.

Valnet J (1982): *The Practice of Aromatherapy.* Saffron Walden, Essex: CW Daniel.

Vickers A (1996): *Massage and Aromatherapy: A Guide for Health Professionals.* London: Chapman and Hall.

Walsh D, Morrissey M (1998): Aromatherapy: an approach to managing symptoms of stress. *Mental Health Nursing* 18(5):23-7.

Wing DM (1998): A comparison of traditional folk healing concepts with contemporary healing concepts. *Journal of Community Health Nursing* 15(3):143-54.

Yerby M (1996): Managing pain in labour. Part 2: non-pharmacological pain relief. *Modern-Midwife* 6(4):16-8.

General Appendices

APPENDIX 1

Australian Nursing Federation Policy Statement: *Complementary and Alternative Therapies*

It is the policy of the Australian Nursing Federation that the use by nurses of complementary and alternative therapies which are deemed appropriate by the client, the client's condition situation and the nurse is supported. These forms of therapy may be provided to clients across the life-span, within the continuum of wellness/illness and for psychological and physiological comfort and wellbeing.

ANF believes that the nurse provides a service which embraces the concept of total health care. The nurse has knowledge and an ability to function in a role which encompasses:
1. promotion of health and the prevention of disease
2. restoration and maintenance of optimal health and health education
3. empowerment of individuals to take responsibility for their own health care needs
4. assisting individuals to achieve a dignified death.

The effectiveness of these roles may be enhanced through the use of complementary and alternative therapies, in addition to, or in place of orthodox medicine (see attached glossary).

PRACTICE ISSUES FOR NURSES

- The therapy/therapies should be included in a plan of care.
- Ingestible products should not be given as part of the therapy.
- Workplace policies on the adoption of complementary therapies or alternative therapies should be encouraged and developed.
- Consent (verbal or implied) should be obtained before any intervention or therapy is given by a nurse. An explanation must be given to the patient/client before any therapy is commenced. If the patient/client is unable to consent, then relatives may give consent.

- The nurse should also check the appropriate institutional policies relating to client consent. Consent/refusal may need to be documented in the case notes. The entry must be signed and dated by the nurse giving the therapy.
- Consent requirements apply to all nursing interventions or therapies whether labelled orthodox, complementary or alternative.

SPECIALISED FIELDS

The therapies which have come to be known as complementary or alternative to orthodox medicine vary greatly in complexity and thus vary in the education and training required to undertake them safely and effectively.

Some therapies are within the nurse's scope of education and some require additional appropriate preparation. The use of dietary adjustment as an alternative to laxatives; the use of gentle body massage complementary to pain control medication; or the use of warm drinks and music as an alternative to sedation medication are examples of choices of therapy within the nurse's scope of educational preparation.

Specialised techniques and modalities such as acupuncture, acupressure, aromatherapy, hypnotherapy and reflexology should only be practised to the extent of the nurse's specific education in the field through accredited programs.

GLOSSARY

Acupuncture
Techniques whereby needles are inserted into specific sites on the body surface to improve the flow of energy around the body, thus preventing and treating disease and disability.

Acupressure
Techniques whereby finger massage is applied to these same points, combined in shiatsu with general massage.

Alternative medicine/therapies
Diagnostic and therapeutic practices which are separate from, and in contrast to, conventional scientific medicine. The term 'alternative' implies use of these therapies rather than orthodox medicine.

Aromatherapy

A sense therapy using specific patterns of sense impressions to heal imbalances and assist in cure, with oils, vapours and essences as the therapeutic agents.

Complementary medicine/therapies

Diagnostic and therapeutic practices which are separate from, and in contrast to, conventional scientific medicine. The term 'complementary' implies use of these therapies in conjunction with orthodox medicine.

Reflexology

Massage of areas of the feet to treat organ systems with which they are in developmental relationships.

Massage

Any technique in which pressure and touch are applied to the body to stimulate the circulation to relax the tissues.

Orthodox medicine

The aggregate of diagnostic and therapeutic concepts and practices which attempt to adhere to modern scientific principles.

APPENDIX 2

Royal College of Nursing, Australia Position Statement: *Complementary Therapies in Australian Nursing Practice*

INTRODUCTION

Complementary therapies are widely used in Australian society and are acknowledged as making a significant contribution to the health care of Australians (Australian Bureau of Statistics, 1986; Victorian Parliament, 1986; Lloyd et al., 1993; and MacLennan et al., 1996). Consumers are increasingly asserting their rights to choose modes of health care, be informed of health care options and be given informed and unprejudiced information.

Nurses are responding to their clients' needs, and to their own needs for professional satisfaction, by seeking to qualify to use complementary therapies; integrating into practice a range of complementary therapies and advising clients on the appropriate use of therapies. Within a context of complementary care and advancement of practice, complementary therapies are increasingly being considered as within the range of nursing interventions.

DEFINITIONS

Nursing interventions are understood to be 'actions performed by a nurse that will help to achieve a patient outcome that falls within the realm of nursing' (Snyder, 1992:5).

Complementary therapies are understood as therapies used in holistic practice and derived from:

- traditions of healing (e.g. aromatherapy, acupuncture, reflexology)
- therapeutic use of self (e.g. humour, therapeutic touch, validation therapy)
- physical therapies (e.g. massage, hydrotherapy)
- energy therapies (e.g. meditation, guides imagery, music therapy).

Healing is understood to be a process which moves towards order and integration of the whole person incorporating the capacity to adapt or evolve (McCabe, 1995). The process can be supported in various ways or suppressed.

Holism is understood to be a tendency in nature towards creation of complex and integrated wholes and systems whose behaviours cannot be reduced to those of smaller units (Capra, 1982:21). Holism is the philosophical framework of holistic nursing which addresses the whole person as a living system interdependent with his/her social and environmental systems.

Complementarity is understood to represent the dual nature of matter as either particle or energy wave. In people it represents the indivisible physical and energy/spirit aspects of being (Rogers, 1970; and Newman, 1986). Complementarity offers an emerging theoretical framework for a holistic approach to health and healing.

Complementary care is understood to be an approach to health care which recognises the principles of holism and complementarity as they apply to health, nursing, healing and therapeutic interventions.

Royal College of Nursing, Australia believes that:
The nursing profession has the right and obligation to interpret complementary therapies within the context of nursing theory and practice.

The nursing profession has a responsibility to provide evidence for efficacy of complementary therapies employed as nursing interventions.

Registered nurses are professional health care providers who are qualified to make appropriate judgements decisions and recommendations to their clients regarding the nursing care to be provided including the application of therapies in the complementary mode as nursing interventions. The use of complementary therapies in nursing practice by registered nurses, either as private practitioners or as employees, is appropriate where the nurse:

- has a qualification appropriate to nursing practice and is competent to practise accordingly;
- practises within the scope and context of the legal framework as set down in Nurses Acts; professional standards; guidelines of regulatory bodies and the policies and protocols in work settings; and
- practises within the limits of their knowledge and skill.

RATIONALE

The basic principle of complementary therapies is the recognition that the healing response is an innate capacity of living beings (McCabe, 1995). Holistic nursing theory embraces the concept that persons are indivisible wholes in all aspects of being—physical, emotional, mental, spiritual, social and environmental (Dossey et al., 1988).

Holistic nursing theory recognises that nurses interact with persons at all levels of being. Complementary therapies can provide a focus for the active promotion of health, healing and wellbeing and the empowerment of people to participate in the healing process. The concept of complementarity supports the nursing profession's role in providing an essential level of holistic, person-centred care which complements physical, disease oriented care.

Royal College of Nursing, Australia recommends that:
Policies should be developed by employers in consultation with nurse practitioners, to provide guidelines for the use of complementary therapies in their facilities. Guidelines should include reference to the:

- consent and documentation processes and procedures
- qualifications and competency of practitioners
- parameters of accountability of practitioners and employers
- identification of which complementary therapies may be practised in the workplace
- consultation and collaboration with experts in the field including, as appropriate indigenous healers (World Health Organisation, 1978).

Nurses practising complementary therapies should obtain personal professional indemnity insurance. It should be noted that the existence of a workplace policy on use of complementary therapies and the holding of insurance by an employer may not necessarily be adequate liability cover for an individual nurse.

The nursing profession should increase its research activity in all theoretical aspects of complementarity to increase knowledge and enhance understanding of the efficacy of complementary therapies.

Royal College of Nursing, Australia resolves to:
- support the profession and its endeavours to integrate complementary therapies into nursing practice
- encourage complementary therapies education providers to seek recognition of their courses through the College's accreditation program
- encourage discussion on the place of complementary therapies in nursing education and of healing frameworks into nursing theory
- assist nurses who may wish to include complementary therapies in their practice to inform themselves about their legal, educational, ethical and professional obligations.

REFERENCES

Australian Bureau of Statistics (1986): *Australian Health Survey.* Cat No 4311. Canberra. ABS.

Capra F (1982): *The Turning Point: Science, Society and the Rising Culture.* London: Flamingo Collins.

Dossey B, Keegan L, Guzzetta C, Kolkmeier L (1988): *Holistic Nursing: a Handbook for Practice.* Rockville: Aspen Publications.

Lloyd P, Lupton D, Wiesner D, Hasleton S (1993): Choosing alternative therapy: an exploratory study of sociodemographic characteristics and motives of patients resident in Sydney. *Australian Journal of Public Health* 17(2):135-144.

McCabe P (1995): Exploring the phenomenon of healing: healing as a health capacity. *Australian Journal of Holistic Nursing* 2(1):13-24.

MacLennan A, Wilson D, Taylor A (1996): Prevalence and cost of alternative medicine in Australia. *The Lancet* March (347):569-573.

Newman M (1986): *Health as Expanding Consciousness.* St Louis: Mosby.

Rogers M (1970): *An Introduction to the Theoretical Basis of Nursing.* Philadelphia: FA Davis.

Snyder M (1992): *Independent Nursing Interventions* (2nd edn). Albany NY: Delmar Publications.

Victorian Parliament Social Development Committee (1986): *Inquiry into Alternative Medicine and the Health Food Industry.* Melbourne: Government Printer.

World Health Organisation (1978): *Primary Health Care: A Report of the International Conference on Primary Health Care.* Alma-Ata. USSR, 6-12 September.

APPENDIX 3

Nurses Board of Victoria: *Guidelines for Use of Complementary Therapies in Nursing Practice*

INTRODUCTION

In recognition of the increasing interest shown in complementary or alternative therapies by the general community, and by a significant number of nurses, the Nurses Board of Victoria provides these guidelines which aim to assist in establishing appropriate standards for the use of complementary therapies. The Board's Guidelines provide a basis for the formulation of policies, procedures and protocols for particular practice settings.

A number of complementary therapies such as massage, have been elements of nursing care for many years, while others, like aromatherapy and acupuncture, are relatively new to the Western health system.

'Complementary therapy' is a broadly based term generally used to describe any approach to healing which lies outside the therapies used as part of 'orthodox' medicine. Complementary therapies are often combined with mainstream health care to achieve a more holistic and integrated approach.

In relation to nursing, complementary therapies are defined as those approaches to healing which are chosen and used in nursing practice to promote health, healing and quality of life and are congruent with the aims, practice and scope of holistic nursing care.

In the provision of holistic care the nurse recognises the consumer's physical, psychological, social, cultural, environmental and spiritual needs and expectations.

The Guidelines apply to all nurses and midwives currently registered in Victoria, including those who incorporate complementary therapies into their practice, or who work as complementary therapists.

EDUCATION

Nurses are responsible for acquiring and maintaining their complementary therapy knowledge and competence, and for being aware of the limitations of their knowledge and competence in relation to complementary therapies. Nurses function within the limits of their education and competence and consult or refer where necessary.

Complementary therapy courses should be carefully selected, bearing in mind the following factors:

- the quality of the education, e.g. course curriculum materials, duration of the course, and teacher qualifications
- accreditation or approval of the course by a relevant complementary therapy professional organisation or statutory authority
- qualifications conferred, and the level of practice for which the course is recognised
- recognition of prior learning
- availability of ongoing professional development

FRAMEWORK FOR PRACTICE

The use of complementary therapies by nurses and midwives occurs within the framework of holistic practice. Within a holistic framework the nurse may utilise knowledge of complementary therapies to support the healing abilities of the individual. Nurses incorporate knowledge of complementary therapies into their practice in a variety of ways.

- ask about, and document the use of, complementary therapies by consumers as part of health assessment and history taking.
- recognise the implications of the combination of complementary and other therapies with other therapies including Western medicine
- consult with, and refer to, appropriate health care practitioners
- utilise selected complementary therapies as either an adjunct to, or main modality within, their nursing practice
- use complementary therapies according to their level of knowledge and competence (competence ranges from a basic level, with guidance from an experienced practitioner, to an advanced level practitioner).

The nurse respects the consumer's individual needs, values and culture and their right to make informed choices in relation to the use of complementary therapies. The nurse acts to support the consumer's choices within the bounds of safety and the consumer's rights and responsibilities.

SELECTION OF COMPLEMENTARY THERAPIES

The nurse considers the following criteria when selecting a complementary therapy for use in her/his practice:
- consumer choice and health goals
- available evidence of the safety and efficacy of the therapy based on empirical data and research
- suitability for the needs of specific consumers
- compatibility with holistic nursing theory and practice
- respect for, and acknowledgment of, the consumer's culture and belief system
- type, level and quality of initial and ongoing education available
- access to mentors, and experts for professional support, consultation and referral networks
- availability and nature of complementary therapy professional organisations
- consideration of other staff/consumers in the area where complementary therapies are in use
- sensitivity to the consumer population, other health professionals and managing bodies
- legal and ethical implications for use in nursing practice.

COLLABORATION, CONSULTATION AND REFERRAL

Collaborative practice refers to a model where each practitioner is autonomous when dealing with issues relating to their professional area of practice, but respects, communicates and discusses management with colleagues, consumers/patients.

Nurses using complementary therapies establish appropriate consultation and referral networks to facilitate access to experts in the field, and communication between health care professionals and the consumer. Where appropriate nurses discuss the use of complementary therapies with other health care professionals in the interest of consumer safety.

PROFESSIONAL CONSIDERATIONS

Standards

A registered nurse using complementary therapies practises in accordance with the *Nurses Act* 1993, the Board's *General Statement for Nurses Undertaking Clinical Practice/Procedures* 1999, and the *Code of Practice for Midwives in Victoria.*

The nurse takes into account the *ANCI Code of Professional Conduct, the Code of Ethics,* and the *ANCI Competency Standards.* The nurse practises in accordance with these standards and codes whether she/he works principally as a nurse or complementary therapist. Professional codes and standards of relevant complementary therapy associations are considered where they exist.

Legislation and regulations

The nurse, practising responsibly, understands and adheres to current legislation and regulations relevant to the use of complementary therapies. These include, but are not limited to:

*   *Nurses Act* 1993
*   *Drugs, Poisons and Controlled Substances Regulations* 1995
*   *Therapeutic Substances and Goods Act* 1989
*   *Australian and New Zealand Food Authority Act* 1991
*   *Health (Infectious Diseases) Regulations* 1990 No 85
*   *Traditional Chinese Medicine Act* 2000

Professional indemnity

Each nurse should ensure that there are satisfactory arrangements in place for professional indemnity insurance. It is recommended that a nurse who practises complementary therapies regularly confirms the extent and nature of such cover as it relates to complementary therapies.

Informed consent

The informed consent of consumers is sought and documented. Where a therapy lies outside usual nursing practices, the nurse ensures that the client is able to make an informed decision to accept or refuse the therapy and documents the client's decision.

Documentation

Adequate, accurate and contemporary records of complementary care are maintained.

GLOSSARY OF TERMS

Alternative
In the past 'alternative' referred to those systems of medicine, such as traditional Chinese medicine or naturopathy, which may have been chosen as an alternative to orthodox Western medicine. In fact, where an unorthodox system is the first choice for care, orthodox medicine may be used as an alternative.

Healing
Is an innate capacity that supports the move from disease or imbalance to balance and integration. Healing can be supported or suppressed, and is dependent on the internal and external resources available to the person at the time.

Holism
Recognises the tendency in nature to form complex and integrated wholes and systems that are interconnected with other systems. A whole system is capable of complex behaviours that separate parts of the system cannot produce.

Integrative
The combination of orthodox and complementary therapies to achieve a holistic approach to healing.

Modality
Describes a method or manner of treatment.

Natural therapy
Is another term used to denote a therapeutic practice that supports the healing process by methods other than pharmaceutical medicines and surgery.

Orthodox
Currently accepted conventional health care. The terms 'Western', 'orthodox', and 'allopathic' are often used interchangeably to refer to currently accepted medical practices. In a similar manner 'alternative', 'natural', 'integrative' and 'complementary' are used to refer to healing systems that are not orthodox.

These guidelines are to be read in conjunction with:
- General Statement for Nurses Undertaking Clinical Procedures
- ANCI Competency Standards for the Registered and Enrolled Nurse
- ANCI Code of Professional Conduct for Nurses in Australia

- ANCI Code of Ethics for Nurses in Australia
- Code of Practice for Midwives in Victoria
- Complementary therapies in nursing — Nurses Board of Victoria briefing paper.

Index